The Gifts Animals Can Give

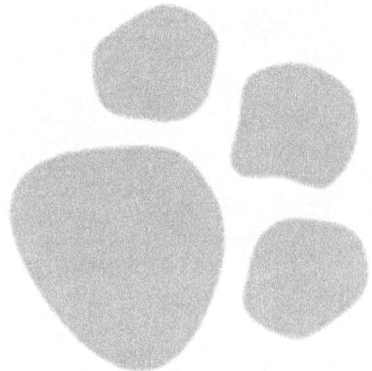

The Gifts Animals Can Give

Harriet May Savitz

iUniverse, Inc.

New York Bloomington Shanghai

The Gifts Animals Can Give

iUniverse books may be ordered through booksellers or by contacting:

iUniverse
1663 Liberty Drive
Bloomington, IN 47403
www.iuniverse.com
1-800-Authors (1-800-288-4677)

Because of the dynamic nature of the Internet, any Web addresses or links contained in this book may have changed since publication and may no longer be valid.

The views expressed in this work are solely those of the author and do not necessarily reflect the views of the publisher, and the publisher hereby disclaims any responsibility for them.

ISBN: 978-0-595-50251-6 (pbk)
ISBN: 978-0-595-61435-6 (ebk)

Printed in the United States of America

Dear Reader:

In this book, I come to you more vulnerable than I have ever been. Always accustomed to the protection of traditional publishers, access to their editors and marketing departments, this time I choose to come to you through modern technology, but also with the creative integrity of the "old days." When the fate of the book was in the author's hands from beginning to end, with all its blemishes and all its truths. When mistakes were made and forgiven because the creativity deserved that forgiveness. There is no guarantee that The Gifts Animals Can Give will sell, bring me fame or deserve more than just one satisfied reader. But that is enough for me. To write a story that is read. Again. And again. A writer can have no greater joy.

Most Respectfully
Harriet May Savitz

P.S. There are no photographs of my pets in The Gifts Animals Can Give. This will free you to see the faces of the pets you love.

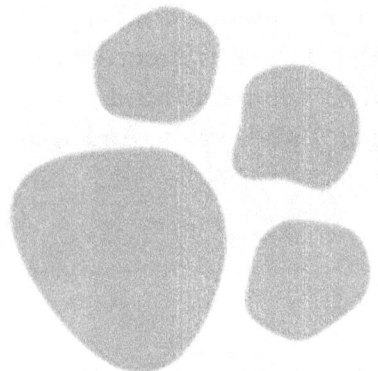

To my family, Beth, Todd, Steve and Liz, including grandchildren Jake, Jenny, Ryan and especially Ben, who wanted to know about all the animals I ever had. This one is for you Ben. Now you know.

H.M.S. 2008

Contents

Acknowledgments

Morrie Berman

Ira M. Blatstein

Edward B. Davenport

de Grummond Children's Literature Collection

Cindy and Kevin Fornino

Carol Franzwick

Linda Hadley Hoffman

Arlene Smith

Ferida Wolff

Belmar Wall Animal Hospital

You know how important you are to my writing world.

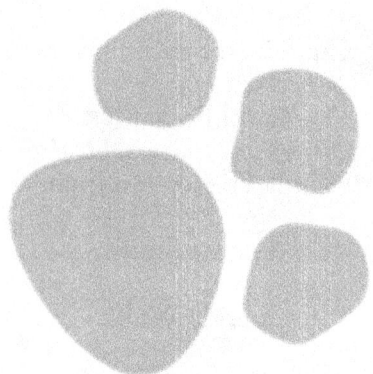

Introduction

My brother was born when I was eleven years old. Until then, I was an only child. I didn't have a close friend, so there were many lonely hours to fill. Whenever a dog or cat lost his way or found himself without shelter, he would follow me home from school or from a walk or from the park. It was as if I had a sign pinned on me, "I am looking for a loving playmate. Come home with me and be my friend."

It didn't seem polite to refuse a lost animal a meal and a warm place to sleep for the night. Just for the night, of course. After all, we lived in an apartment house and everybody who lived there knew we were not allowed to keep pets.

But one night usually turned into two, and sometimes three. Just as we were beginning to be friends, just as I was growing accustomed to being greeted at the steps when I returned from school, with the wag of a tail or a loving meow, someone in the apartment would complain. Someone would tell the landlord.

The story was always the same. I would return home from school and my companion, my delightful pal would be gone.

"We gave the dog to someone who had a big backyard," my mother would tell me, trying to soften the blow.

But I kept bringing strays home. Even for a little while, they provided companionship and I learned how quickly animals could entwine themselves into my life, as if they had always been there.

A lonely day was never quite as empty with a dog's nose nuzzling against my knee, begging for attention. A cat on the bed at night, even if just a stray passing by, purring me to sleep, softened the harsh memories from a day at school. An animal never told me my clothes were not stylish as my classmates did, or that I was too shy as some of my teachers believed. Animals accepted me just as I was and seemed to think everything about me was perfect.

"Some day I'm going to have as many animals as I want," I promised myself. Years later, when that some day arrived, I did.

Now I am 74 years old, and find my animal companions are more necessary to my life than ever. I'd like you to meet my animal friends as they came into my life, and some, as they left. Share with me their gifts. After you've met them, I promise the world will seem less lonely for they will remain in your heart as they have in mine.

1

The Grump

o o o o o o o o o o o o o o o o o o o o o o o o o o o o o o o o o o o

The Grump was a tough taskmaster. He had been on the streets and knew his way around. One look at me, and the Grump realized I needed to learn a few things about dogs. He became my teacher.

One of the qualifications I had to have in a potential husband was that he love pets. But one doesn't just find out such information immediately. During the dating time with my husband-to-be, I told him about my lifelong love of animals. I didn't ask him the important question about his feelings, because I truly liked him very much, and was afraid he would give me the wrong answer. Then I would have to leave. It was that important to me. After knowing each other several weeks, he knocked on my door. I was still living with my parents in a "No Pets Allowed" apartment. In his arms was a little puppy. It seems he couldn't stand it one more minute, my not having my own pet, and so he bought me one. Do I have to explain the commotion that ensued? I was delighted, my parents were frantic, the young man was confused, not knowing the apartment's rules and regulations. However it was agreed by all that I could keep the pet for awhile, at least until we were married which was also agreed upon that evening. And then we could take the dog with us. The end was not a happy one. The landlord found out and we had to find another home for the dog. But it would be the last dog I would ever give away.

As soon as we bought our own home, we went to the animal shelter to find a pet. Of course I wanted all of them at once, the cats peering back at me, the kittens, the puppies and the grown dogs that begged for love. One

1

dog just sat there staring into my eyes. There was no mistake about it. He was a mutt without an inch of pedigree. He looked as if he had been through too many rainstorms and too many owners, though he was but a puppy himself.

"Pedro is not too friendly," the woman warned me. "He doesn't bite but he doesn't make friends easily. It might be difficult to place him."

I knew what that meant and it seemed so did the dog. He nuzzled his nose toward the cage so that I could pet him.

"Well, that's new for him," the woman said. "He usually doesn't get affectionate with anyone."

My husband and I had one infant at home in our new house. We had some serious thinking to do about bringing a new dog home, especially one that had the reputation of being difficult. There were other animals available; beautiful, friendly, happy, eager. This dog with unattractive brown hair was none of those things and yet, I felt he belonged in my life. I wanted to give him the love he had missed before. Perhaps on his good days, he might offer my family some love in return.

As soon as we took Pedro home, it became clear that his devotion was confined to our immediate family. Everyone outside the front door was his enemy and once they opened the door they had to immediately prove that they offered friendship. As master of his house, he growled automatically at the turning of the knob on the front door. "Who could it be?" he seemed to question. "Have they come to hurt my family?" Pedro's upper lip curled and a nasty expression encircled his face. He was always on the job.

"It's O.K. Pedro," someone from the family would assure him. His brown eyes would turn sweet, his lips into a soft welcome. But he didn't fool anyone, certainly none of my friends.

Whenever I told others, "He's such a sweet dog," my friends would stare at me. Were we both talking about the same dog, the one who had the habit of nipping at neighbors heels when they came to visit, the dog who wouldn't let just anyone in the house, especially those he had doubts about. And Pedro had doubts about everyone. He was certain the mailman was depositing something dangerous into our mailbox each day. The newspaper boy became an instant enemy the moment he stepped into the driveway. The milkman never stood a chance. Pedro didn't like his truck. In fact, he didn't like all trucks, uniforms, people with loud voices, and especially strangers.

Gaining Pedro's approval was no easy matter. A pat on his head or a gift of a bone wouldn't do it. Neither would talking to him in dog language. "Sit," went unnoticed. "Stop," was ignored. He could not be bribed or fooled. If he liked someone, he barked his welcome and then disappeared into his nap area. But if anyone was on his suspicion list which was very long and growing, he'd stand his ground by the front door while one of the family tried to persuade him that though he was in charge of entrances and exits, we were in charge of him. Of course it was far from the truth.

"Just let us in, Pedro. You liked us yesterday." There would always be someone coaxing by the front door. And then with a frown, once in, "Why do you put up with that dog, anyway?"

That was a difficult question to answer. Pedro was disagreeable and even a bully. He disliked most everyone he didn't know and just tolerated those he did. But he loved his immediate family and we knew it. We understood the outside world had treated him cruelly and he could not forget nor forgive it. Sometimes though, he got his enemies confused with his friends.

Grandmom Sarah came to baby-sit occasionally. Pedro and she had a mutual understanding. She did not go into his territory. He did not go into hers. If Pedro didn't trust her, the feeling was mutual. But one day their paths crossed in the backyard. Grandmom gave Pedro a piece of her mind about his rude behavior and how she thought their home would be much better without him. No one was certain what followed after the lecture, neither was very clear about it, but Grandmom wound up with a nipped finger and said she never wanted to see that dog again. From then on, Grandmom and Pedro were never in the same room. Pedro seemed to agree it was best for both of them.

"Why do you put up with him?" became the question most often asked.

It was a question that I couldn't answer and even if I did, no one outside the family would understand the answer. Pedro offered us a different side than he offered elsewhere, one without violence, without bad temper. He was our protector with a commitment that never weakened. When one of our children started down the stairs head first, it was Pedro who grabbed hold of his diaper with his teeth and pulled him away from the steps. It was Pedro who stood in front of anyone in the family when a stranger approached. He guarded our front door, our back door, our windows. He lived for the family.

"Is Pedro in a good mood today?" a friend would ask before visiting.

"He seems to be," I would answer.

But was he? He looked as if he were, sitting there peacefully in his favorite spot, window gazing from the couch. His ears were tucked back, his tail curled beneath him, a sign he was relaxed.

"Are you a good dog today, Pedro?" I would ask.

The tail wagged, the ears flipped up. He turned my way. "Of course I'm in a splendid mood today," he seemed to say. "It's the people out there who are causing all the trouble."

Pedro's gift to us was unconditional love. It was wrapped in a package few would recognize. He loved our family, especially the children. They could do anything to him, break all his rules, touch him unexpectedly, play with him endlessly, and he would just gaze at them lovingly, not a growl from his lips, nor a complaint. The tail would wag and he would look at me as if to say, "It's just fine. Don't worry about it. I have everything under control. After all, they are just kids."

Pedro was my first dog. He taught me about loyalty to family. His was undaunting.

2

Miss Respect

○ ○
It isn't easy being the first. First dog. Now first cat. But the difference here was that I always thought of having my own dog. A cat never occurred to me. I thought they were nice creatures in someone else's house. And then one day, Tawnie came to my house.

All my daughter wanted for her seventh birthday was a red bicycle. Naturally, as loving parents, my husband and I bought one for Beth and kept it hidden in a nearby shed to surprise her. But when Beth was asked to make a wish at her birthday party, you can imagine our surprise when she wished for a kitten instead of the bicycle.

This wish was made in front of 20 neighborhood children and it is well known that birthday wishes cannot be denied. While the birthday cake was being cut and devoured, my husband rushed to the Animal Shelter around the corner. He returned with a beige kitten with light blue eyes and a haughty expression. We named her Tawnie because of her coloring, bits of beige mixed with white. She was so tiny; she fit into the palm of one hand.

We had a difficult task ahead, one might say impossible, to introduce the mighty Pedro to this infant kitten. While the dog was locked up, we let Tawnie run around the house, sniffing under things, poking her nose in dark corners, investigating our home as if she were deciding if it were suitable. We directed her to the kitty litter pan and let the children take turns holding her. But I did warn my daughter that this experiment might not work out. Pedro would have to decide if it did. He was not good at sharing, especially his family and household. It would be his decision, with a little help from those who loved him.

Tawnie came to her own decision about Pedro and their living together. She certainly knew how to use her claws and her mouth. Even when Pedro rushed into the room, even as I held Tawnie tightly and felt her tremble, I also felt her strong claws dig into my skin. She spit. Pedro growled. She stretched her claws in his direction. He showed his teeth. He protested, sulked, barked into her face. Tawnie responded by stiffening her back and puffing her tail in a sword-like fashion. It was obvious though Pedro was shocked, insulted, stunned, and disgusted, he had met someone as stubborn as he was and as determined to have her way. Later, they had a showdown by the front door; a place Pedro considered his domain. Tawnie struck his nose with one clean swipe. It was a bulls-eye. Pedro yelped, jumped, threatened and cried. From then on he avoided any confrontation and whenever in her company, he showed appropriate respect.

Tawnie immediately delivered her message to every member of the family and to all visitors in one way or another. Respect. She demanded it from everyone. She would not tolerate rough treatment or a lack of sensitivity. She used her paws or a sharp meow to keep us in place.. And she reminded me how important respect could be in one's life. As a mother with two growing children of my own, the one consideration I demanded was respect. Tawnie and I were on the same page when it came to behavior.

Because Tawnie was my first cat, she had to teach me everything. I must admit she had patience. I had never owned a cat when I was a child. Now I had one who kept telling me what to do and how to do it. She taught me the basics about what she expected in her new living quarters. No, she wouldn't eat her food on the floor. Perhaps other cats did, but Tawnie insisted eating on the dishwasher, out of Pedro's reach. She would sit there at mealtime and wait and meow. Quite loudly. Consistently. If the food bowl was set down in another location, she would not approach it. "Meow. Meow." Until her message was understood. Her bowl of water had to be changed twice a day or she wouldn't drink it. "Meow. Meow" by the water dish. The poor dear had a lot of work to do when it came to communicating with me. I was accustomed to a dog's bark and knew what it meant, but unfortunately a cat communicating was not adequate at the beginning. Tawnie did a lot of meowing. She had a favorite chair to sit on which happened to be my favorite chair. So we had to share it. And sometime during the night, Tawnie felt the need to lay on my chest with cat whiskers resting on my chin. It was necessary for Tawnie to adjust her sleeping habits at my insistence.

Whatever made me think cat food would be accepted by Tawnie as the only food. It was quickly rejected for any table food available, especially chicken, hamburger and tuna fish.. Eventually I even learned never to interrupt Tawnie's nap.

Tawnie took naps in the most unlikely places. Not only on my favorite chair, but on the kitchen table, on my pillow in bed, in a box wherever a box was put, and on my desk. She also enjoyed eating my plants, no matter how I tried to put them out of reach. They suffered greatly, and eventually only those that were not to Tawnie' taste survived. A hunter always, Tawnie slipped into her cat mode at the sight of a bug crawling on the floor, a moth flying near a light bulb. Around and around her head would move, following it, trailing it, waiting, always waiting to give a quick swat of the paw.

Gradually the family grew to know what was acceptable to Tawnie and what was not. Rude behavior was not. Though she loved my daughter Beth and spent a good part of the day sleeping on her bed, or waiting for her to come home from school, she would not tolerate Beth's habit of tweaking her nose whenever she passed. Tawnie never let her get away with it without a reprimand. A paw with claws withdrawn, slapped back. Hard. "Mom, Tawnie hit me," Beth would complain. "What did you do to her?" I would ask in return. Children now grown into adulthood recall Tawnie as a strict disciplinarian who made certain the rules of polite behavior were observed.

Rule #1. Nobody pulled her tail. The tail that communicated her moods and swished back and forth if she grew inpatient was not to be touched by the hands of a human being. Rule #2. No one could pick up Tawnie in a sloppy or sudden manner. Both hands please and gently. Rule #3. She insisted on promptness. When the alarm clock rang, telling us it was time for school and work, she immediately jumped on each bed, licking faces, a rough tongue urging everyone to get up.

"Just one more minute," family members would plead, but Tawnie was not one to bargain. She wouldn't go back to her nap until everyone was awake and moving. Using her bag of tricks, she accomplished her goal.

"Meow. Meow. Meow." First into one ear, and then another. Under the blankets with her cold nose digging into flesh. Claws kneading into any exposed area of skin.

But waking us up was just the beginning. Tawnie then followed everyone into the bathroom, watched them shower, brush their teeth, then led the procession down into the kitchen. She insisted that her food be put on the dishwasher first, before anyone else ate, but she waited until they were seated around the kitchen table before she began eating. It was a courtesy she extended her family each morning.

However, Tawnie parted company once nighttime approached. While we were ending our day, she was beginning hers. The mysterious hunter inside her would rise in the darkness. Tawnie could be heard scurrying about in the kitchen, knocking over things. It was her time to explore. She wasn't allowed outside, but there was much to investigate inside. The storage room held dark corners cluttered with shelves. Perhaps there was a mouse lingering. There were the stairs, not as interesting in the daylight but now cloaked with intrigue. What fun to run up and down them when the family was out of the way. Up and down. Up and down. Hour after hour. "Doesn't that cat ever sleep?" someone would complain. "She's doing it on purpose." Her paws, so silent in the daytime, now sounded like elephant's feet.

One cold, wintry night, Tawnie's need for adventure led her into danger. We had opened the front door to let someone in, when Tawnie dashed out. She had never expressed any interest in the outdoors so we were unprepared for her flight into the darkness. We ran after her, but she was faster and played the game of hide and seek much better than we could. Her cat's eyes maneuvered easily as she hid from us. We heard her meow, teasing us with her call, and yet our flashlights could not find her.

After several hours in the cold, we temporarily gave up our search. We kept the light on in front of our house, hoping she would find us again, or we would find her at our front door in the morning. None of us slept well that night. There was always a face at the window looking out, calling, "Tawnie, are you there?" The next morning we searched again, asking neighbors, driving our car slowly down the street. The alarm clock would ring in the morning and we would wait for the cold nose, the licks on our faces. .

Every hour of every day, we wondered what Tawnie was doing out there, how she was surviving. Always in charge in our small world, we feared for Tawnie's safety in the larger one. We called Animal Shelters, told our friends, and put flyers up on trees and poles. Each day we would return home, one of us asking, "Is Tawnie back?"

After two weeks had passed, we had to admit the possibility that Tawnie might never return. But I was not ready to give up. I took the garbage can from the side of the house, stood it upside down, placed Tawnie's favorite tuna fish in a dish on top of it, and waited inside. Each night I changed the food. Each night I hoped to hear a movement against the can. None came.

And now three weeks had passed and we didn't speak of Tawnie any more. It was too painful. I put her inside dishes away and her favorite toy. It was the day before New Year's Eve and we were having a party. We had become so preoccupied with Tawnie's absence, we neglected to make our usual decorations. So the evening before, we all sat around on the floor with signs and magic markers, half heartedly creating happy slogans for the New Year's Eve party. People kept knocking on our door, bringing in their contributions.

It was quite late when we heard another kind of knock. It was more like a tapping sound.

"Who's coming this late?" I thought as I ran to the door.

I didn't expect to see Tawnie hanging on the doorknob, with one paw rapping on the door. Quickly I carried her inside. She was light in my arms, having lost weight. Her hair was matted, her face thin and worried, her eyes watery. Her meow was weak as we fussed over her, warming her to our bodies as she trembled in our arms.

The next day we took her to the veterinarian. He said she was frightened and had gone many days without food, but otherwise she was in good health.

That night, after we had all eaten dinner, we watched Tawnie sit on the dishwasher, cleaning herself. She had recovered her dignity as she cleaned her ears and tail and shined her coat.

Beth passed by and tweaked her nose. Tawnie retaliated with a slap of the paw.

"Respect. Respect," I could almost hear her saying. "I demand respect."

Whatever prompted Tawnie to run away that night never tempted her again. She lived for many long years in our house, and the door opened many times, but she never ran outside.

And we never stopped giving her respect.

3

Living in The Moment

o o o o o o o o o o o o o o o o o o o o o o o o o o o o o o o o

We were a middle class family with an upper class dog. With her, we had a touch of class. With us, she became one of the gang.

For the first time in many years, we were a dog-free family. Pedro had passed on. We tried to convince ourselves there were benefits to being dog free. No dog to walk. No reminding someone, "Did you take out the dog?" No asking, "Did you feed the dog?" No dog bones lying around the house to trip over. No fleas itching the dog and ourselves or expensive flea medicine. And certainly no loud barking all the time. We considered ourselves strictly a cat family now as we entered our mid-life years .Until the day we visited our local pet shop. Actually we were there to buy one of our cats a toy.

"It's wonderful not having a dog," I reminded my husband as we glanced over at the dogs in pens waiting to be purchased. And the expense of it all, I thought as I walked closer to one of the cages. I'm not certain how it happened. I don't recall that it was intentional that I stood there, squealing the fateful words, "Oh, what a precious dog!" As the statement rushed from my lips, I knew I was in trouble.

I had my nose pressed against the cage and the nose of a small dachshund pressed back. She looked like a long hot dog. Her color was cocoa brown. She had a cone shaped head, and a large chest. Her eyes were hungry for love as she put one paw against the cage door and entered my heart.

"Isn't she beautiful," I sighed.

"And expensive," my husband added with some reality. "Who would spend that kind of money for a dog?"

Our dogs always had come from the Animal Shelter. "This one's a real pedigree," I explained, defending the dog who continued to look up at me as if pleading, "Come on. You can convince him. You know we have to be together."

"Only $150.00," the store manager told us, sensing he had a potential sale in his hands. "A real bargain. They go for much higher. We're having a sale today." The manager must have seen us weakening. He continued his sales talk. "The Dachshund is considered the national dog of Germany. In central Europe it was once used to hunt badgers. It has a good sense of smell."

My husband looked at me in disbelief. Were we actually discussing the possible purchase of this dog? We certainly couldn't afford $150.00 for a pet. There were more important things to buy, like shoes and clothes for school. And a new sofa for the living room. The outside of the house begged for a painting and the front door should have been replaced a year ago. This dog deserved to belong to a family that could afford it, in a house with a large backyard, maybe even a servant or two to take it for walks. It deserved a fancy dog collar, perhaps one made of rhinestones and a fancy coat to match.

Cocoa was nibbling my hand. In my mind, I had already given her that name. Her soft kisses were delivered to my fingers. And those brown eyes wouldn't let go.

A dog coughed in a nearby cage.

"Some of these animals aren't even healthy," my husband warned.

More reason to rescue her, I thought. Cocoa wagged her tail. It was a long, skinny tail, darker brown then the rest of her and certainly of lesser weight. She was sitting down, her plump stomach resting against the floor of the cage, one paw rubbing the bars.

"I'd never pay $150.00 for a dog," my husband announced as he rubbed Cocoa's nose and received a generous tongue scrubbing in return. He lingered five minutes too long, long enough for her to spin her magic web about him.

One hour later, we walked out with Cocoa in our arms. We did not try to explain to one another how we had convinced ourselves this dog was meant for our family and that we could not live another day without her. Even if we had to give up the new couch. We decided later, when she sat in our living room like some precious statue, that we were just hypnotized by her beauty.

A visit to the veterinarian the next day brought shocking news. The newest member of our family had a disability, a degenerative spine that would probably grow worse as she grew older. It would shorten her lifespan.

"I would return her," the veterinarian said. "The pet shop owes you one healthy dog for that kind of money. They'll give you a refund or another dog."

Cocoa was unmoved by the news of her disability. She seemed completely happy with her new home and her new family. Her tail wagged constantly. She welcomed visitors, was interested in everything about them and loved everyone instantly. Loving was her specialty. All I had to do was look at her and she made me happy. It was as if she knew she had a limited time and she didn't intend to waste one moment of it brooding about life's problems.. When she wasn't wagging her tail, she was playing ball with the children or playing catch the cat.

Each day that passed, though we didn't speak of it, we knew our chances of returning her grew slimmer. While I should have been thinking about doing just that, lifting her up, putting her in the car, and driving to the pet shop, I was studying her face, and thinking, if I were an artist, I would have captured it in a painting. Dark eyelashes over large brown eyes. Bright eyes, shining, full of fun. A thin long nose and soft ears that hung soulfully low.

"She's smiling," I told everyone one day. "She actually smiles."

I couldn't give that smile away, or all that beauty. It just didn't matter that the smile cost us $150.00 or that it had come in a slightly damaged package. We had a bit of sunshine in our house and it was named Cocoa.

Cocoa grew longer and fatter. The more pounds she put on, the more difficult it was for her to walk because of her spine and the problems it presented. If the children or I noticed that she needed help, we would just lift her up the stairs, or on to a chair, or wherever else she wanted to be. She was very polite about such things, waiting for someone to discover her plight, and didn't mind at all when she was carried. The pedigree in her appreciated the special attention.

If she ever had a bad day, Cocoa never let us know it. She woke up every morning happy, and greeted us as if we had been on a vacation for at least a week, when all we had done was sleep through the night in our bedrooms. Even if we went out on an errand for an hour, she would be there when we returned, jumping around with excitement as if she couldn't bear another moment without us. When visitors arrived, she would sit nearby and listen attentively to the conversation, as if she were part of it. It didn't matter to Cocoa if it were raining outside, or the sun was shining. She had a perpetual smile on her face. She was just a happy dog. And somehow that happiness was contagious. It was difficult to hold on to a dark mood with Cocoa doing all kinds of tricks to get our attention. If she ever did something wrong, which was seldom, none of us could reprimand her. It was impossible to call a time-out on a dog whose entire purpose in life was to entertain and offer affection.

We bought her a red sweater for the winter. Anyone who had the pleasure of seeing her stroll down the street in her new attire had to stop and bend down, way down, to pet her. She was irresistible.

'What a beautiful dachshund," we often heard as Cocoa paraded up the block.

She made it easy for us to forget she had a disability. She was seldom ill. And she never complained. The veterinarian explained to us whenever we took her for a check-up that her condition was worsening. She wasn't in pain but some day she might be. It was like a shadow over our heads and yet when we experienced Cocoa's zest for life and her ability to enjoy every day, it seemed impossible that anything would daunt her spirits.

We pushed the fearful thoughts aside. Cocoa helped us do it. She rolled on the ground until one of us rolled with her. She loved the snow and dug her way through it. If it was deep enough, she would actually disappear and often we would have to run out and rescue her from drowning in a snowdrift. And she never tired of playing with children. If there was a ball rolling around, she was running after it. If someone was riding a bicycle, she might be in the basket in the back. If anyone was taking a sleigh ride, they were holding Cocoa in their arms as they whizzed down the hill. And a red wagon. Nobody ever got into a red wagon without Cocoa sitting in front. It was as if she knew she must cram everything of life into a small space because her time was quickly running out.

The veterinarian never understood why we had kept Cocoa when we knew from the beginning that she would cost us a lot of time and money in the end. And she did. It seemed every week there was something we weren't sure of and had to check into. A back leg or a front leg. More vitamins. Possible therapy. New medications. It was money we could probably have spent well elsewhere. Sacrifices were generously made. Sometimes it was opening up a piggy bank to pay the vet bills. Other times it was doing without a dinner at a restaurant or seeing a movie. But none of us minded or gave it serious thought. Cocoa deserved the best we had to offer. And she gave us her best, every day.

In later years, our family often gathered around to reminisce about our beloved dachshund. There seemed so much to remember. The gifts she had given us were abundant. Her ability to enjoy life to the fullest was the greatest gift she left with us. Cocoa took the cards life had dealt her without bitterness or complaint.

She made every day count.

Questions from My Pets

"What's to eat this morning?"

"Did you forget my treat today?"

"Are you ready for our walk around the block?"

"How about some playtime?"

"Who's that knocking at the front door?"

"How about changing the menu once in a while?"

"Could you move over so we can both sleep on the pillow?"

"Do you really have to sit on *my* rocking chair?"

4

The Listener

∘ ∘

I never thought of having a turtle for a pet. In fact, I never thought of having one in my house. Turtles lived outside. Red Fox, a box turtle, did not ask to come inside, but once he did, he had no intention of moving out.

Thirty-five years ago, my husband and son visited the mall to pick up some school supplies. They returned with a box turtle with orange-red eyes, a tank, turtle food, a water pan and directions on how to take care of a pet box turtle.

"Who's he?" I asked, not remembering him on my list of things to buy.

"Red Fox," my son answered.

"How long is he staying?"

"Don't worry," my son answered. "I'll take care of him."

I knew what that meant. My son always promised to take care of our pets. He never did.

The next day, as I cleaned Red Fox's large tank, I had the opportunity to study him. My past experiences with box turtles had always been as they passed in the road going or coming from some secretive place. Sometimes I would discover them near a stream or by some woods, hidden like a large rock. They didn't seem to be interested in me and I felt no interest in them. Red Fox and I looked upon each other now with the same disinterest.

Tawnie expressed some fascination with the new addition to the family. She sat in the tank, staring down at the box turtle that had his head buried inside his shell. Red Fox had no inclination to come out for many days, though it was not his hibernating season. We left food, cooked chop meat, cut up tomatoes, bits of dog food and chopped corn to tempt him, but the box turtle left them untouched. If this represented his attitude about his new home, we clearly had been rejected.

There was nothing endearing about the box turtle that appealed to me. In fact, when describing him to my friends, I used the term "ugly, positively ugly." Red Fox had a dark shell, a scaly leathery neck, orange-red eyes that looked more blood-shot than any I had ever seen, and a mean expression. I could tell even with his head stuck in his shell that he wasn't a pleasant guy and had no intention of making friends with me.

Most of Red Fox's world lay in his tank. He had a small piece of wood, a rock, a water pan, and a hut. The tank rested on a bureau in front of the window where the sun splashed on it. Nobody can live in our house without at least a good morning from me. So I said, "Good morning, Red Fox," each time I walked into my son's room. Red Fox never acknowledged my greeting. The weeks and months passed. The most we could say for Red Fox was that he was there. Silent. Lifeless. Like a rock in a corner of his tank with no interest in the outside world, or for that matter, his inside world. Occasionally we might catch him stretching his long legs as he walked toward his water pan or eventually, his food. But once we walked into his room, he quickly tucked his head back into his shell and turned into an immovable object again. It was as if he were telling us, "I have no intention of making friends. So beat it."

It was definitely a one way relationship for many months. I always greeted Red Fox in a friendly manner. At least he couldn't say I wasn't trying for a better relationship. "Good morning," I said while I made the bed, or watered the plants. "How are you doing today?" I'd ask as I got together the laundry. Of course I didn't expect an answer, but a head sticking out from his shell would do. One day Red Fox surprised me. He stretched out his neck and looked up toward me, staring as if he were saying, "Good morning," in return. Soon after he greeted other members of the family in the same way. It was as if he had made up his mind that since this would be his permanent residence, he was going to make the best of it.

Red Fox eventually created his own schedule. He liked to sunbathe in the mornings, take a bath sometime during the day, eat a couple times a week, though during the hibernation season, he could go much longer without food, stretch out his scaly legs when he rested on his rock and sometimes, with supervision, take a stroll in our backyard.

The years passed. "How long do box turtles live?" I asked one day.

"Very long," my son answered. Of course at the time I didn't know box turtles could outlive their owners.

Ten years passed and Red Fox and I had come to an understanding. Since I was the one who cleaned out his cage, gave him fresh water, tended to his meals, it seemed only natural that he and I should connect in a special way. I discovered Red Fox was an excellent listener. Everyone in my family had schedules and appointments and play dates and school dates. But Red Fox's calendar was open. He was always willing to come out of his shell, stretch his long neck, turn in my direction, and level his red-orange eyes on me as if I were the most important person in the world. Gradually, I confided in Red Fox my fears and my dreams. I felt he understood. When someone has been with you ten years on a daily basis, it is only natural to feel a certain trust.

Though he seemed perfectly content in his large tank, we would take Red Fox for walks, sometimes in the room on a rug. Red Fox would scurry into dark corners, into closets, under the bed, as if he were playing a game. Though slow in the tank, he was surprisingly fast out of it. He had a sense of direction only known to box turtles, and he surprised us by repeating his journey to the same closet, or the same hallway. We would turn him around to see if he would become confused, but he never did.

In warmer weather, we took him outside. We were very careful watching him, for the outside world stirred the wanderer in him. Up one hill, around the rocks, through a trail, into a puddle. Discovery upon discovery. And if we looked away for a moment, he would disappear, camouflage himself. We would panic, thinking he was lost forever. And then the grass would stir as if he knew we needed help. He always made certain we found him.

My son Steven, who was now in college, had little time for Red Fox. I, on the other hand, found myself with an empty house. The turtle and I had much in common now. He had lost his playmates. They had grown up and gone away to school. I had lost my children in the same way.

"Is he still alive?" Steven's friends would ask when they returned to visit.

"Look for yourself," I'd say.

So Red Fox became sort of a celebrity, just by being there, through one generation and then another. Also he became a teacher. He taught me every day as I peered into his tank. His world wasn't large, but he seemed content with it, busy in his own way. Sometimes he sunbathed on his rocks, other times he buried himself in his hut. Often he lay in his water dish, cleaning himself. He had interest in everything around him. And in his silence, he often offered comfort. Once I thought him ugly. As years wore on, I found beauty in his red thoughtful eyes, his leathery neck, his protective shell. And I never needed a calendar to tell me of the change of seasons. Red Fox offered his service. For years, I depended on my bread box to tell me when spring was approaching. The sun splashed on the bread box a certain way and even if snow was on the ground, I knew spring was heading my way. The bread box told me. Now Red Fox told me when a season was coming to an end or about to begin. All summer he was busy, active, marching back and forth in his tank, standing on his hind legs to get a better look at things, meditating on his rock. Occasionally he made his way beneath his water bowl and carried it on his back around his tank, as if he were rearranging furniture. Of course the water spilled over the tank and I had to clean it up. I think he did it intentionally to get my attention.

As soon as the weather grew cold, I would hear familiar noises in his tank. Red Fox was shredding the paper on the bottom of the tank and making himself a hut. Sometimes I would think he was too early or had gotten mixed up with the months because the weather was warm, but soon he would prove right and the cold would descend on us. He always knew when winter was approaching.

Red Fox taught me the benefits of hibernation in the winter, to feel it's o.k. to stop the running and the doing. Slowing down was permissible in his world and he taught me it could be in my world also. Why run out in the cold when one could rest on the bed, read a book, meditate, or dream.

Years later, as a widow, I made a decision, soon to be reversed, that it was time for me to sell my house. There would be no extra space in my new apartment, especially for a large tank. The family met and made the decision while the box turtle listened as usual, his head turned upward. Red Fox would go to a zoo. He would have a wonderful time discovering things, and he would be with his peers. Why not let him roam free. Certainly a box turtle must have other ideas about the way he would like to spend his life.

The morning of his departure I sat on the bed next to his tank and looked over at him.

"Today's the day," I told him. "You're on your way to a new life."

I always spoke to him in that fashion, as if I were in conversation with another person Usually he faced the window and the sunbeams coming through it, but this time, he turned and looked directly at me, his orange eyes holding mine for one long moment. The message he sent through them could not be misunderstood.

"You've got to be kidding," they seemed to say. "I've stuck with you through thick and thin, through screaming kids and family ups and downs and now you're going to stick me in a zoo, with strangers. Would you do that to any other member of your family, abandon them like this?"

I wouldn't tell too many people what happened next, because who would believe me, that when I picked up Red Fox and lay him on my shoulder and stroked his shell in a final goodbye, who indeed would believe that he stretched out his arms and legs without fear, that he nestled his head into my shoulder, that I felt his hug and his love and that when my son arrived, after traveling an hour and a half, after taking the tank and Red Fox and packing them into his station wagon, that I ran outside and yelled, "We can't do this. He's part of our family. I'm keeping him." And then I decided to remain in the house that I loved so that both of us would have all the room we needed..

"Is Red Fox still alive?" friends still ask Thirty five years later, he certainly is.

5

The Slob

o o o o o o o o o o o o o o o o o o o o o o o o o o o o o o
*Puff was quite proud of her tail. She held it high when she walked
by, shaping it into a thick plume. It did not matter to her that the
tail was covered with food and anything else that happened to be
available.*

We were attending the Strawberry Festival, my daughter, my son and I.
Every year we visited the spring celebration on the grounds of the Friends
School. What better way to celebrate this exit from winter than with
games of chance, plants for sale, and the aroma of baked goods filling the
air. It was a time for families to get together with old friends after a long
winter, and exchange news.

Every year we would play the games and always win a goldfish. We
could count on one sure thing at the Strawberry Festival. Everyone won a
goldfish. Then we would buy a bowl, some fish food, and our Strawberry
Festival fish would live out its days in our kitchen, in a sunny corner, out
of harm's way.

This particular year, we didn't win a fish, though we tried. We stayed
longer then usual trying, watching others win, but it was not in our destiny to take a goldfish home with us. Much of what was being sold had
been bought by others by the time we finished trying to win a prize. There
were a few boxes remaining and our curiosity prompted us to poke about
in them looking through some discarded books. One box had nothing in
it but a small patch of fur. Ear muffs, I thought as I bent over to pick them
up. Then the ear muffs moved.

The fateful words, "Oooh, what a cute kitten," greeted me from one of my children, who was an impatient teen-ager and until this moment, bored with the afternoon. "It's a Persian kitten."

The woman in charge petted the kitten, now in my arms. "The only one left of a litter," she reported. "She was on the bottom sleeping. To tell you the truth, I forgot she was there. Isn't she beautiful though? She is not a purebred, but look at that tail."

The woman picked up the tail straight in the air. "That tail is twice her size," she said proudly.

It was true. The tail was more like a plume on an ostrich, thick and filled with gray, orange and red colors. It *was* twice the kitten's size.

The ball of fur yawned in our faces, then returned to sleep. She didn't seem worried about her future as was the woman trying to sell her to us. She also was not impressed with any of the people around her.

"She really deserves a good home," the woman said, getting ready to leave.

When my husband and I had brought Pedro home, we were a young couple newly married, with tiny tots in tow and a new house. Now we were settled in middle age with two lively teen-agers seldom home. We had an adult box turtle as well as a senior cat. Since Cocoa passed on over one year ago, there was no dog. Life was comfortable. Tawnie enjoyed her kingdom. It was a one-cat house and she liked it that way.

We later blamed it on the fact we didn't win a fish, that we brought home the Persian cat whom we promptly named Puff. "She'll be company for Tawnie," I explained as if that would make sense of it all. "I think cats should be in pairs."

Tawnie had other ideas. She took one look at Puff and disappeared into the closet for two days, only coming out for the necessities of life. When she finally appeared in public again, she bitterly meowed her disapproval. "How could you destroy my perfect world," she seemed to blame me as she looked down at the small ball of fur sleeping at her feet.

"Treat her like a sister," I suggested to Tawnie. "Sisters can be wonderful. You'll see. It's not good to be an only cat. You don't get a chance to share. This way you'll never be lonely and you never can tell what excitement Puff will bring into your life."

Tawnie just stared at me with her large blue eyes. She didn't buy my story. Instead, she spit in Puff's direction, her tail straight in the air as a warning when she walked by. She chased Puff away from her toys, her food, her favorite sleeping spot. She refused to eat with her, play with her, or to acknowledge her existence in any friendly manner.

To make matters worse, Puff had personal hygiene habits that repulsed Tawnie and disappointed us. She was not a clean cat. She didn't seem concerned that her fur got matted and dirty, that she carried all the dust in the house with her. Whenever she ate, bits of food clung to her face and the thick fur around it. Sometimes even her ears carried the remains of dinner. When she would turn around from the water or food bowl, her tail often managed to dip into it and take whatever she was eating or drinking. Tawnie's face puckered with disapproval as Puff walked by, smelling from dried food.

But in spite of the fact she was often a walking garbage can, Puff's gift to the world was her beautiful tail. It rose like a submarine periscope. As she grew older, the tail grew thicker, and its colors changed in the winter to hues of gray and yellow, in the spring to the brighter orange and reds. She displayed it proudly, caring little whether it had been cleaned recently. When she had time for a bath, she'd take care of it. There was no rush. Maybe today. Maybe tomorrow. Certainly it wasn't a reason to delay a nap. In fact, there was little in life she found imperative. A good meal. A nice drink of water. A perfect nap. Someone stroking her. Life was good.

Puff could boast of little else beside her tail. She wasn't too bright. When she used the kitty litter, she would sit in the wrong direction. Her head and front paws dipped into the litter while the part that belonged there, hung off the kitty litter box onto the floor. We tried training her, reminding her. We'd turn her around, congratulate her when she succeeded, reprimand her when she didn't. But Puff was unmoved by our training sessions.

Eventually Tawnie realized she had to take matters into her own hands. Otherwise Puff would infect the entire house with her germs. Tawnie took over Puff's bath time. Her face showed the distastefulness of the job as she cleaned Puff's ears, around her face, up and down the long tail. She'd look toward me as if to say, "Well, someone has to do it."

Puff was also clumsy. Cats are usually graceful, light on their feet, able to jump from and to high places. Not so for our dear Puff. If she jumped from a chair or a table, she usually misjudged her landing. We would hear a thud, a thump, a crash, as she brought something down with her.

Tawnie never let these errors go unnoticed. "Are you sure she's a cat," the blue eyes asked as she inspected the disaster area.

Perhaps it was all the fur or the thick tail twice her size that kept Puff off balance. It could also have been her weight. Puff's favorite pastime was eating. She was on time for every meal, and when Tawnie didn't finish her food, Puff was there cleaning up the dish. Her needs were simple. She loved to sleep, and only then did grace enclose her as she tucked her tail around her body and curled her paws inward.

But she had little interest in us as a family. She happened to live with us but that was an accident. She didn't care to nestle on our laps nor did she pay much attention to our household schedule. Yet she was quite agreeable if we picked her up, moved her, carried her around. She was almost like a piece of furniture that could be placed anywhere without responding. Her meow was soft, faint, as if it were hidden in all that fur. But since she had little to say, it didn't much matter how quietly she said it.

Puff's favorite dinner was corn on the cob. We discovered she liked it one night, when it lay uneaten on a dish, waiting for dinner. There was Puff, taking action, sitting on the chair as an adult would, her front paws stretched upon the table, one paw turning the corn while her sharp teeth bit off the remaining kernels. The next time we had corn on the cob, we cooked Puff her own portion. Sure enough, when it cooled, she was on the chair. We rejoiced. At last we found something Puff could do. Whenever anyone special attended dinner and we wanted to impress them, we just cooked corn on the cob. Puff never disappointed us. Word spread throughout the neighborhood children. "Are you going to have corn tonight, Mrs. Savitz?" I was often asked. "Can we watch Puff eat it?" Puff became a minor celebrity on the block. Of course we would have preferred that she perfected her kitty litter performance instead. Someone was always cleaning up after her.

And someone was also always carrying Puff with them. My daughter, after a bad day at school, would call, "Where's Puff," and then finding her, carry the limp cat to her bedroom. I would find them sprawled out together, Puff resting on her stomach. Or my son, after tossing the basketball in the driveway, would grab Puff and charge up the steps. Puff would accompany him while he changed clothes. Perhaps that was her greatest gift, keeping us company. Her serenity was comforting.

It was during this time that my husband became ill and Puff's companionship needed. He was home from work for a long time, with little to do. Being a very active man, he found it difficult to do anything but read or watch television. That's when Puff became the teacher, and my husband the student. Relaxing was Puff's specialty. She could fall asleep anywhere, on a chair, on the floor, hanging over a table, half off a window ledge. We had to be careful not to step on her because her sleep was deep. Tawnie heard noises a block away, a thunderstorm hours before it arrived. Not Puff. The storm could be overhead, crashing down upon her. It wouldn't disturb her slumber.

"That cat doesn't care about anything but sleeping," my husband said one day. "I sure wish I had her attitude. Nothing worries her. Nothing keeps her up at night. Nothing even keeps her awake all day." Puff was sleeping on his shoe as he spoke.

Being unable to work was difficult for my husband. The doctor told him it was urgent that he relax. It would be weeks before he could return to his job. An active man doesn't settle down easily. That's when Puff went into action, as much action as a non-active cat could manage. Wherever my husband sat, Puff sat with him. Not just with him, but on him. As if to keep him down. She was heavy enough to succeed. Usually disinterested in all of us and our comings and goings, now she appeared alert and on duty to one person in the house. Relaxation was her specialty. If she took my husband in hand, she might even convince him a daily shower wasn't necessary. Leave the dirty dishes on the table. Forget about combing your hair. Come join me in a sunspot and snooze away the day. Or better yet, let's have a treat to eat. Or sit by a window and daydream. There are a million ways to waste away a day and Puff knew every one of them.

She and my husband became inseparable. When he arose, Puff was there. When he ate breakfast, Puff accompanied him, lying on the kitchen table. Usually he would scold her and chase her off. Now he not only ate his cereal, but offered her some milk in a small bowl near him. When he made his tuna fish sandwich at lunch, he left some for her in a saucer. They sat together watching television. She sensed when he was tired, when he was restless, when he was sad, and when he was scared. And then she would cover him with her heavy body as if to soothe away his fears.

Often, I would find him sleeping next to her on the couch. Or while holding her on his lap. She somehow made his convalescence easier. Her calmness, her contentment, her easy going manner, was contagious. The two of them became devoted companions. If my husband sat talking on the telephone, Puff slept on his lap. If he read the newspaper, chances were Puff was snoozing between the pages. When my husband returned to work and to his schedule, Puff returned to her schedule. But at night when he slept in bed, she always curled herself about his feet, doing what she did best. Being there.

6

The Boss

o o o o o o o o o o o o o o o o o o o o o o o o o o o o o o o o
We were grateful to Sam that she allowed us to live in her house. By no means was it ours. The moment she moved in, each room, each cupboard became part of Sam's domain.

Loving an animal is easy. Taking charge of its life, being responsible for its safety, and ultimately deciding when it must be put out of its misery are much more difficult decisions. After Cocoa, when she silently looked toward us for help as her pain grew unbearable, we agreed we had enough for awhile. We needed time to grieve for our dear friend and we also needed time to forget the pain we felt when making the decision that she could no longer live a life of quality and dignity. In other words, we were finished with dogs for awhile.

A neighbor raised Beagles and called us down to see the litter. Going was our first mistake. Picking up Samantha in our arms was our second one. She was a beagle, all ears, black and white, with dark eyes.

Of course we instantly forgot about all the reasons we didn't want another dog, and took her home. To a house with two cats and one box turtle. We weren't worried about the box turtle's reaction, but Puff and Tawnie had little opportunity to meet dogs since Cocoa was gone, other then watching them through the window and thinking how lucky they were to have the window between them.

At the beginning, Samantha was smaller than each cat and so she was no threat. In fact, it was the contrary. Both cats ganged up with a few swipes to Sam's nose and ears to keep her in line and remind her that a cat's claws can be mighty weapons.

Sam was brought up by our cats. She bathed herself when the cats did. She ate with them when they did. She sunbathed with them and played with them. There were times when we were afraid she might forget she was a pure bred beagle.

That was a laugh. Samantha never forgot and never let anyone else forget. She wore her pedigree in her walk, in the expression on her face and in her hearty beagle bark. "Ahhhhooooooo." That bark traveled down the block, around the corner, as far as the shopping center two blocks away, when she had the scent of a rabbit. Any rabbit who heard her beagle warning was already packing its suitcase and heading out of town.

Everyone in the family has a Samantha story. She lived sixteen years with us and left her adventures as part of our family history.

The food stories: Samantha was a human vacuum cleaner when it came to dining. She had little respect for the command, "Down, Sam. Get away from the table." Down when there was steak for dinner? Down when there was a sweet smelling sandwich or her favorite hot dog? Sam could leap faster than the human eye could follow, on to a table, right past my nose, from the floor to the chair, away with the steak, before anyone realized the meal had disappeared. Instructions were given to visitors. "Do not leave your food unguarded." Even so, we often heard the frightening query, "What happened to my sandwich?" Eventually we put up a gate blocking Sam at mealtimes. But nothing could block her protests. Every meal was accompanied by the ear piercing. "AHHHHoooooo."

Samantha loved birthday cakes. We discovered this on the first birthday party she attended. We had a wonderful time blowing out the candles and distributing the pieces of cake. Then we went into the living room to open the presents. Unknown to us, Samantha jumped on the dining room table and devoured the remainder of the cake. One would think we would learn from that experience. But beagles are very cunning. She knew we were watching her and so the next time a cake was available, Sam pretended disinterest. She sat perfectly polite with her best manners, listening to the conversation around her, her beagle head turning this way and that. Yawning now and then as if she were ready for a good nap. Not noticing the cake wherever it was. We would in fact, forget she was there. Through the years we learned, never forget Sam. She could be anywhere. It was a perfect record. Over 16 years, one way or the other, the first day or the second, from the top of the table to beneath it, Sam always outsmarted us and never left a cake untouched.

The man who gave us Sam had other beagles from the same littler. "They are all so obedient," he told us, apologizing as if it were his fault. "Why can't you train that dog?" And then he'd come and give Sam a lecture about her behavior. Of course Samantha always snatched his sandwich before he left.

We had occasion to go away one summer and there were no pets allowed at the boarding house. We decided it would be a wonderful opportunity to send Samantha to camp. Not only would she have a vacation in the mountains but the owners assured us Sam would return to us better than ever. They were accustomed to training dogs.

"I want that dog to sit when I say sit, and stop when I say stop, and I don't want him to jump on my kitchen table any more." Those were my instructions to the owner of the camp when I left.

Our beagle was only there two days when we received a phone call. It seems that Sam did not like camp. She expressed her disapproval by barking her beagle bark throughout the night and day until all the other dogs were unsettled and barking with her. She never stopped. The owner admitted he had never heard a bark so loud and so constant. In fact, he complained he had a big headache and he attributed it to Samantha. He concluded his life would be much better without her in his camp. We had to leave our summer place and travel to the mountains to pick up Sam and then find a dog sitter for her in our home. That was the end of Sam's formal behavior training. Or perhaps that was the beginning of ours. Sam's way.

Burying the Treasure Stories—Sam was a true beagle. She always had the scent of something and she always was burying a treasure. Most of her treasures consisted of socks. She'd wait until nighttime, watching us undress. "Don't forget to put your socks in the laundry," I'd caution. But

Sam knew someone would forget, or there would be a sock dangling from the laundry basket. It was gone in a minute. None of us had matching socks because of Sam's obsession. She hid them everywhere, under the couch pillows, behind the sofa, under our bed pillows, in her sleeping basket. Now the problem with the buried treasure was that Sam resented anyone threatening to discover what she had hidden. If we happened to sit unknowingly near a buried sock, Sam would smile. At least it looked like a smile. Actually it was the expression before she jumped toward her treasure and destroyed the composure of anyone sitting near it. A leaping growling beagle can do that to someone. "How cute," a visitor would comment. "The dog is smiling." One of us was sure to hurry the visitor to another location.

Running Away stories—Sam was always running away. She never got lost and certainly had no intention of leaving home permanently, but it was the adventurer in Sam that got the best of her now and then. She would run past our legs out the open door. One day, she actually jumped from the kitchen table, out an open window on the first floor. We didn't even know she was gone until a neighbor walked up the street carrying her in his arms. Sam was young then. As she grew older, it became more of a challenge. Samantha would run down the street, sniffing the ground as if a rabbit were underneath the cement, and we'd call behind her, "Sam, come back here." She probably interpreted those words as, "Sam, run as fast as you can," and she did. And we'd run after her. Sometimes we would be running in our pajamas. Neighbors became accustomed to our attire. Other times in the winter without a coat. For Sam on the run was a maniac on the loose. Freedom was ahead. Behind her were strangers who were nothing but a nuisance in her quest for a good rabbit hunt.

Walking Sam Stories—Sam loved her daily walks. Actually she took us for them. She was strong and she would pull on the leash until we dragged after her. During the day she went about her business quietly sniffing the ground, interested in every crawling thing. Only at night, or at 3:00 in the morning when she stood at our front door letting us know there was an emergency, would Sam suddenly take to the cement and vocalize her feelings. "AHHHHOOooooo." It echoed up the street. Lights would flicker on in houses. I knew the entire neighborhood would be waiting for me the next morning with their complaints.

"Shhh. Sam. Be quiet," I'd plead.

"AAAHHHHOOOooo!!!" she'd respond with the same disdain she displayed toward any command.

Garbage Can stories—Sam had a love affair with garbage cans. She couldn't pass one by without tipping it over, and then sorting through it. Samantha usually managed to secure something chewable. She made her rounds every day, from the bathroom to the kitchen. Eventually we had to enclose the kitchen garbage can beneath the cabinet. When Samantha learned to open the cabinet door, we had to put on a lock. We never doubted that eventually she would learn how to unlock it.

Sam's close calls—A three-pound box of chocolates she devoured one night and sent us all to the emergency room of a veterinarian hospital. The doctor attending couldn't believe she was still alive.

The German Shepherd who lived across the street was feared by everyone. He got loose periodically. Samantha, on one of her free runs, delighted in tormenting the Shepherd when he was chained, running back and forth just out of his reach. One day Sam thought he was tied on his usual chain and he wasn't. Both of us ran for cover that day.

Sam's IQ stories—Samantha understood everything. Every conversation. To a point where we had to spell. And then she learned to spell also. If she heard, "Let's take Sam to the Vet," she was gone, under a bed where we couldn't get her. If she heard, "Don't let Sam see we're having steak for dinner," she was there, under the kitchen table, refusing to budge. "I have to give Sam a P I L L," would send her fleeing into another room.

Sixteen years. That's a long time for a dog to be part of a family. We forgot what life was like without Sam. Eventually, she ran the house. She ran the cats. She ran everyone and everything that came into her space. But she did it with class. She always wore that haughty expression on her face as if she expected us to know better. Certainly she would want what was on our plates rather then what was on hers. Certainly she would prefer an old ratty sock then a new toy. Certainly she would have to dump over every garbage can for there might be a bone forgotten in there. Certainly she would want to sleep on the bed, on a pillow right next to us, with her cold wet nose pressed against our skin, rather than in her sleeping basket, all alone. And yes, please cover her up with a blanket to keep her warm.

Sam resented only one thing. Being treated like a dog.

"Why don't you just put the dog outside in a dog house?" someone suggested. "That way you'll have some peace."

We couldn't because Sam didn't think of herself as a dog. If we left the house on vacation, Sam usually accompanied us. She expected that. If she didn't, arrangements had to be made and not just casually. We had to leave someone in charge Sam approved of or else she would cause havoc.

Sam had her duties and she took them seriously. She baby sat with any children when they were on the premises and she made certain they didn't wreck the house or ruin her nap time. She kept me on my toes in the kitchen where she was concerned with menus, and never failed to greet my husband when he returned home from work.

We loved Sam unconditionally. Her personality, like a mosaic, brought something different every day. She dug her way into our lives and our hearts. We never thought of letting go. She'd be with us always. She didn't make always, but she did survive 112 dog years.

Occasionally when I go up into the attic where we retired Samantha's sweater, her sleeping basket and her favorite socks, I hear her calling out AHHHHOOO! As if to let me know somewhere she is still on the hunt. And I smile.

Pet Volunteering

A working neighbor might need you to pet sit for awhile.

Veterinarians might need help in the care of their pets.

There are pet shelters in need of volunteers,

Lost animals in need of foster homes.

Groups are constantly having fund-raisers for homeless animals

Even the simple gesture of

Feeding the outdoor birds and

Squirrels can give purpose to the day.

7

The Peacemaker

o o o o o o o o o o o o o o o o o o o o o o o o o o o o o o o o o o

Two dogs? It never occurred to me that I would bring another dog into the house. But destiny decided otherwise. There was enough love for both.

Ten years into Samantha's life, Mogul stepped on the stage. I always believed I could have two cats, even three, and be able to handle the situation. But dogs are a different matter. One has to walk a dog, play with a dog, and if the dog was like Samantha, watch a dog. It becomes a full-time job. I thought I could not handle two dogs living in my home.

My daughter, Beth, acquired a dog. She was living away from home in her own place and she missed not having animals. A friend living out in a rural area brought Beth the news her sheep dog had a litter. The puppies were part sheep, part shepherd. I went with her to pick out her dog. There were other puppies available but I remained strong. No, I did not want two dogs in my life. The puppy Beth took to her apartment was beige and white with strands of silver. I had to admit the dog had a unique look.

Beth was away at work much of the time. Mogul kept himself occupied by chewing up her slippers and socks, her pillows and whatever he could find lying around the house to keep him busy. He minimized his boredom by destroying her bedroom.

Whenever Beth visited anywhere outside of work, Mogul traveled along as her constant companion. He grew accustomed to eating corn flakes on the road, sitting in the front passenger seat of Beth's car, finishing up his meals of left-over sodas and French fries. He became the darling of the single set and quite the party dog. If there was a beach party, Mogul sat comfortably on a blanket listening to the conversation. If it was a house party, Mogul had his share of potato chips and a soda to fill his stomach. If it was a long car ride, Mogul sat up front, in the passenger seat. But always he was close to Beth.

Mogul was a snuggler. Whenever Beth got into bed at night, Mogul hopped on her stomach and nestled as close as he could. He perfected the hug and fell asleep that way, both paws around her shoulders. Alone most of the day, he treasured their being together at night. He was there to comfort her, take away her aloneness and always make her feel needed. For Mogul needed her love as much as she needed his.

He was a happy dog. He loved everybody. He hugged everybody. He was willing to eat whatever was put in his dish whether it be tacos or pizza. Mogul was a people person and when he came to visit our house, which always agitated Samantha, I would tell Sam, "Be nice to your cousin, Mogul."

Mogul had just turned one year old when Beth decided to go away on a skiing trip without him.

"Would you just take him for a short time?' she asked. "He'll be so lonely if I have someone he doesn't know take care of him."

So Mogul came for a visit. The two cats and the box turtles didn't mind at all. Samantha was outraged. She bullied Mogul, bit him on the ear, would not allow him near her toys, especially her socks. But Mogul didn't care. He accepted Sam's behavior with his usual good humor and found a pillow to chew on instead. Well, what's a pillow I thought? It's only for two weeks. Because of his good nature, Mogul made the best of it. He attached himself to me, keeping me company in the kitchen while I cooked, at my writing desk while I worked. Samantha had no interest in such petty devotion but Mogul thought it his duty that no one should be alone for long. His soft silver hair would rub against me sometimes during the night as he walked by the side of the bed to let me know he was there.

When Beth returned from her vacation, she presented an idea. Mogul was spending too much time alone and she couldn't be with him as much as she liked. She realized a dog could be limiting for a single woman, especially when she worked full time.

"Look how happy he is here with you," she said. "And all your animals love him."

"Absolutely not," I replied, knowing exactly where she was heading with this idea.

"Well, then I think I'm going to have to give him away," my daughter responded. "But it will break my heart. I'll put a notice up at work. Could he stay with you until I do? It won't be long. I promise."

"Just for a little while," I reluctantly agreed.

Mogul remained for seventeen years. How could we give away a dog that actually made us look good for the first time? As if we knew how to train a dog.

"Sit Mogul."

The dog would sit.

"No, Mogul."

The dog would listen.

"Come here, Mogul."

The dog would come.

And then there were the hugs. Every time we went out and every time we came home. Mogul would stretch his long golden paws and wrap them around our waist as he stood on his hind legs. Mogul was the perfect dog. Well, almost perfect.

He had one very poor habit that could not be broken. He loved pillows. It reminded him of his single days back in my daughter's bachelor pad. He chewed them up as quickly as we bought them. Bed pillows. Couch pillows. Feathers flying in the air. Samantha loved when Mogul was caught and punished, which was usually a stern, "No Mogul." Unlike Samantha who didn't care in the least about a rebuke, Mogul took it to heart. He would hide beneath a bed, or behind a chair, looking as if his heart were breaking. But he was addicted and he couldn't break his habit. We couldn't estimate how many pillows Mogul devoured in his seventeen years.

Chewing pillows wasn't dangerous but swallowing panty hose was life-threatening. Mogul, when left alone for too long, regressed to his old free-swinging ways. One day when we were absent he swallowed a whole pair of panty hose. It didn't take long to see he was in distress. An emergency visit to the vet, an emergency operation and $350.00 later, the panty hose was freed from its entrapment.

Because Mogul came along in Sam's old age, it seemed our beagle grew to enjoy his company. It was nice to have another dog around to take the heat off Sam when she got into trouble, because she knew very well, as perfect as Mogul appeared, one day there would be a pillow forgotten and the feathers would fly. They became the odd couple, inseparable and yet so different in nature.

It was Mogul who helped fill the emptiness when we lost Sam to age and illness. When we returned home that day, Mogul instinctively knew it was his house now. And his job to take care of it. Because of our grief, we left Samantha's sleeping basket out for a few days, thinking perhaps Mogul might use it now. Mogul never did. Perhaps out of respect for his old friend. Now as the only dog, he became more assertive, more in charge. And even more loving.

Aside from his pillow fetish, Mogul was an easy dog. We could leave him in the house with all the garbage cans filled and come home to find them just the way we had left them. We could leave him for long periods of time and never worry about his having an accident on the rug. Now and then, we would forget to lock the back outside gate and Mogul would get out. But unlike Sam, he circled the house and barked at the front door.

There was a gentleness about him. He never bared his teeth or growled or showed any kind of distemper. He didn't have changing moods as Sam had, or a touchy temperament. Mogul always had a good day, until the day I was in jeopardy. That day Mogul nearly sacrificed his life.

An Akita dog got loose and followed us down the street while we were out for a stroll. I only heard the Akita's feet hitting the ground behind me, but it sounded like horses hooves. I ran for refuge into someone's front yard, but the Akita was fast and determined. He charged into the yard and into me, setting me off balance. Mogul stood in front of me, fighting it out with the Akita. People ran out to help us cautioning me to stay away but how could I? My dog was fighting for his life and for mine. Mogul was no match for the larger dog but kept fighting, dodging like a boxer in the ring while I screamed frantically. People around us reached out with brooms, trying to get the Akita's attention. Exhausted, the Akita finally went on his way. When it was over, Mogul was badly bitten over every area of his body. We found out later the Akita had killed a German shepherd by breaking its neck only a few weeks earlier. It took Mogul a year to recover. In a way, that day, he became not only my dog, but my hero.

When I became a widow living alone, Mogul became my companion. One winter night, we went outside in the backyard, both of us not realizing the snow had become much deeper then we thought and the wind much more violent. Mogul ran down the back porch steps and I after him. Both of us fell into the snow and neither of us could get up. Here we were but a few steps away from the porch and unable to reach it again. I remember sitting there in the snow, the wind stinging my face, and all the tears that were left over from losing my husband spilled down my face. In another time and another place, I could have called my husband for help and he would have rescued me. But there was no one to call. He wasn't here any more and that reality hit me hard that stormy night. For a moment I didn't think I could get up. I looked around me. It was late at night and all the lights were closed in the surrounding houses. It was so still except for the roar of the wind. Mogul stood in snow that imprisoned his legs. He looked at me as if to say, "It's up to you my dear lady. Because I can't do a thing." I don't know how I did it, digging him out, pushing him toward the steps, pleading with him to cooperate, resting, pushing, crawling to outwit the wind. Later, inside the warm house, Mogul and I sat in the kitchen. I drank some hot tea and he some warm soup. "We did it," I told him proudly. "All by ourselves, we did it." It was then for the first time, I truly believed I could go on without my husband. With Mogul by my side, I would not be alone.

8

The Pianist

o o o o o o o o o o o o o o o o o o o o o o o o o o o o o o o o

Music can be appreciated by anyone who wishes to be included. Especially a cat.

Before I tell you about Bradley, I must tell you about the meaning the piano had in our lives. The first piano I remember in the family was when I was very young. I was at my grandparents' house. They had a tailor shop and not much money. They lived next to a railroad track and I cried from fright every time the train went by.

But on the bright side, they had a piano in their living room. I don't know who used it. There was a stool in front as if it expected someone to come play. I don't recall any of the other furniture, but I remember the piano.

I received my first piano when I was ten years old. It came from a cousin in Philadelphia. My mother immediately sent me for lessons. I hated the lessons, but I loved sitting at the piano. I decided I might as well practice because you just couldn't sit and stare at a piano. It expected something more of you.

The piano accompanied me when I married. We had it refinished and painted white. My children took piano lessons. They didn't like the lessons either and found any way to get out of them.

Especially my son. He showed up at his lessons without shoes.

"I won't give him his lessons unless he arrives on time," the piano teacher said when the baseball season arrived. "And with shoes."

The calls were frequent. The lessons continued.

For a few years, the piano grew quiet. The children were grown and too busy elsewhere. I only played to entertain myself. Until Bradley came along. He came to us from a friend. People always thought of us when they had a litter. "Oh, the Savitz family will want one of these kittens," they must have said to one another.

We were sitting around playing with Mogul at the time when in walked my husband carrying a kitten.

"Ed's cat had a litter," he said. "He wondered if we wanted this one." Ed was a friend of ours. This one was a pure gray kitten with large white patches down his stomach, around his mouth, and up between his eyes. He looked as if he were wearing a mask. He also looked as if he didn't like us, our house, and certainly not the dog that was licking his paws. Yet he purred deeply into my arms as I asked my husband, "Do we really want three cats and a dog?" I don't remember anyone answering that question. We named him Bradley, after our favorite summer vacation place, Bradley Beach.

Bradley didn't fit in right away. He spent the first few days scurrying into hiding places, as far away as he could get from the dog and the other two cats. His favorite hiding place was behind our vacuum cleaner. He would remain there for days. When he wasn't hiding there, he was on top of the heater. Eventually Bradley found security in another unexpected area. He wrapped himself about an ankle, anyone's ankle, and fell easily to sleep. It was all right at night when we were in bed to have Bradley's warmth about our feet, but during the day, dragging him as we walked became quite cumbersome. .

Bradley felt most secure when he traveled with a dish towel or wash cloth in his mouth. He loved the soft feel of them and couldn't resist stealing one whenever it was possible. I would put a wash rag down on the bathroom sink. Five minutes later it would mysteriously disappear. I would use a dish towel, then hang it on a hook. Later, I would find it on the living room rug. Bradley would clasp it between his back legs and drag it into a room where he would curl his body around it and go to sleep. Other times he just traveled with it hanging from his mouth, dragging it between his legs across the house, as if he had garnered a treasure.

When I sat playing the piano, Bradley would grab his rag and jump up on the piano bench. If I sat there for an hour, so did he with the rag sticking out from his mouth. He had an old face, as if he had lived one hundred years before. I could only wonder what he was thinking. His eyes grew thoughtful as he watched my fingers run up and down the keyboard. It was my favorite time with Bradley for I had his undivided attention. He would poke his nose close to the keyboard, sniffing it. If I remained there for a long time, he would fall asleep resting on his rag on the piano bench. He wouldn't leave until I did.

We thought we knew everything there was to know about Bradley until the night we heard piano playing in the middle of the night. By this time, Bradley had been part of our household for several years. Each of us was asleep in our beds when it began.

"Who's that playing the piano?" I shouted into the hallway.

The entire family made their way downstairs to find Bradley running up and down the keyboard. It didn't surprise me. Now it all began to make sense. Bradley had been studying my piano playing. He wasn't just sitting there passing the time of day. He was taking lessons.

However, I didn't expect the concerts to continue. As they did. Though we appreciated Bradley's new hobby, we had hopes that he might switch to daytime piano playing instead of the middle of the night. But that never happened. From time to time whenever the mood struck him and we were never sure when that would be, our cat would just climb on the piano bench and wake everyone in the house. It was especially distracting when we had overnight guests.

"Did I hear someone playing the piano last night?" a guest would ask.

"Yes, probably," I'd answer. "It was our cat."

There didn't seem to be a further explanation necessary.

However, eventually we had to take action. No one could get a proper night's sleep. Bradley had become an enthusiastic pianist. First it had been five minutes. Then twenty. But when it reached a half hour of running back and forth over the keys, we had to take action. We closed the keyboard at night. I don't know why we thought Bradley would accept such a solution.

"What the heck happened here?" I could hear him protesting as he thumped over the closed keyboard and made enough noise to wake us up anyway. "Why did you have to take away my one moment of creativity?" Thump. Thump. Thump.

It became a battle of wits during the forthcoming years. Sometimes the keyboard was closed. Sometimes someone forgot and it was left open and Bradley went through his concert until we closed it again. We were always forgetting. He was always waiting for us to forget.

Bradley was quite content with his inside world and his rag. He had a short "didn't like" list. On it were plumbers. For some reason known only to our dear cat, when a plumber arrived on the premises, Bradley went into a frenzy and retreated to the heater. This cat that had a face that would frighten a lion, was terrified of repairmen.

One day the plumber, who was fixing a pipe in our bathroom wall, chased Bradley from his hiding place, which at the time was inside a large garbage can. Soon after, Bradley disappeared. Just before the plumber was ready to seal up the hole in the wall, we heard a small scratching sound.

"You'd better wait," I told him. "I think my cat is in that wall."

The plumber peered inside. "There's nothing there," he said.

But I knew there was. "He's in there somewhere hiding. I feel it. We can't seal up the wall until I know for sure where he is."

If Bradley was hiding inside the hole in the wall, I knew there was no way to get him out unless he chose to come out himself. He was not a cat to be bribed. Eventually, the plumber went home with a puzzled look on his face and the promise to return the next day to finish the job. I placed some of Bradley's favorite tuna fish on a plate in the shower. It remained uneaten, the cat unseen. The next morning I received a telephone call from the plumber.

"Is that cat out of the wall yet?" he asked.

"Not yet," I answered.

We left spaghetti in a bowl and some of Bradley's favorite wash rags. We actually had no proof that Bradley was somewhere in the wall except for her disappearance and that one sound I had heard. On the fourth day, with the plumber threatening to leave the job or seal up the hole and "the heck with the cat," Bradley crept out, her tail in the air as if we were the ones who owed him the apology.

His next trauma occurred when we sold the house and had to move. One of our greatest worries was Bradley and how he would accept it. We remembered how he had hidden for two weeks when he first came to live with us. We weren't wrong in our fears. Bradley, who had lived in one house for ten years, who never went outside, who had his favorite place on the heater where he spent his private times, now had to move to a shore house with several floors, winding staircases, skinny hallways and a very dark basement. And to make matters worse, our new home was actually an eighty year old house in need of repairs. Repairmen were everywhere.

Bradley ran into the basement as soon as we let him out of his carrier in our new location. We were relieved because the kitty litter was down there. However, we thought eventually he would come upstairs. He didn't. He found the heater and sat on it for three weeks. I fed him on top of the heater. I gave him his water on top of the heater. And I groomed him on top of the heater.

I called the local veterinarian. "What can I do?" I asked. "He's so angry at me. He spits whenever I go near him. He's blaming me for the move. He'll never come up from the basement.

"Some day he will," the vet assured me. "When he's ready.

Everyone visited Bradley in the basement and talked to him on the heater.

"Are you ever coming up from there?" I wearily asked one day. "You know it's been two months."

Three months to the day, Bradley walked up the stairs into the kitchen as if he had been there all his life. It took the cat an entire year before he would enter the second floor level of the house. Fortunately for him, the piano was on the first floor.

A Week's Worth

Bring a pet into your life.

Spend time with your pet.

Give your pet a treat.

And a check up.

Volunteer to help a pet in some way.

Be pet friendly.

Visit a pet shop and meet other pet lovers.

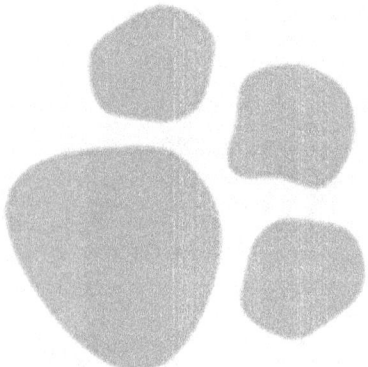

The Later Years

My Worry Page

Will I always be able to take care of my pets?

Will they outlive me?

Who will take care of them if I am not here?

As I grow older, will I make them old with me?

Would they rather be with a young family full of energy?

Am I selfish, at my age, adding a new pet to my family?

If I move, will I be allowed to bring them along, and how could I not?

My Dog

Others might think of my dog as just another dog. Not I. He is my dog. Our personalities are intermingled. I do not know where his begins and mine ends. We have become one.

Without my dog, I would not get up promptly when the morning sun splashes through the Venetian blinds. I could ignore it easily and turn over for 20 more minutes of sleep, or even another hour. There is no job to report to at a certain time. No other person to consider. But my dog knows when the day begins that he must go into the backyard and explore. Chase the squirrels and the cats. Run after a bird. Do his business. He understands I must be out of bed and on my feet so that he might get going. That is his job. To get me going also.

We walk several times a day. Without my dog, I would not notice each tree, each bush, each sweet smelling flower, each unidentified piece of garbage, each person walking toward us, each bird in the bushes, each sudden noise. But with my dog, I notice everything because he does. I do not think I would walk as often or see as much if it were not for my dog.

My dog reminds me to be sociable. Living alone can cause one to forget to be gracious. An unexpected knock at the door often sends me scurrying to another part of my house. Not my dog. He jumps toward the door. Wags his tail. Takes his bone to greet the visitor. Runs around expressing joy. "What a sweet dog," everyone says. And he is. Loving company as he does, he is eager to greet them. No matter what the day. I have never seen him moody as I might be. And he never forgets a repeat visitor. My dog has certain greeting barks for each one. Even the mailman. He goes through all kinds of gyrations when the mail arrives. For within the house and outside of it, my dog is my guardian.

My dog reminds me when it is time to eat. He has two meals a day. Breakfast and dinner. Of course it is understood that he eats first. Or I can have no peace dining. He likes his regular dog food and perhaps a sample of what I will be eating. A piece of chicken. A carrot. Any morsel is appreciated. He is never disappointed by a meal. Unlike family and friends who might not care for my cooking or the meals I create, my dog never complains. Into the bowl. Into his stomach. His appetite often inspires mine. He wags his tail after and licks my leg in appreciation. We understand each other perfectly.

I know when my dog wants me to pet his belly for he turns over on his back, legs in the air, a smile on his face. Reminding me there must be time in my life for a loving moment. He will remain that way for many minutes until I notice. He tells me when he is frightened. He is petrified of thunder storms. His tail goes between his legs and he shivers as if he is in an ice storm. Frantically he will dig into closets, under tables, anywhere he can find shelter. My dog sometimes gets upset with me. Talk of a visit to the veterinarian sets his lips into a sneer that warns of trouble ahead. My dog immediately rushes to the coat closet and refuses to come out. I leave the door ajar. Otherwise he will scratch until there is no door remaining. My dog becomes annoyed if I ignore him. Friends and I might be deep in conversation. He is not included.

"What is your dog doing in the coat closet?" they will ask.

"Sulking," I answer.

Sometimes we just don't like each other. I do not like him when he chews up my slippers, snatches an uneaten sandwich from the table, empties a garbage can, or takes something he knew I treasured and destroys it. He barters. He won't relinquish his prize until I give him a treat in return. I know it is against all training instructions to reward bad behavior but he shredded the rule book long ago.

My dog doesn't like me when I pull at him because I want to go in another direction, when I reprimand him because he is up to no good, or when I wake him up from a sound sleep.

Some say to me, "You could travel. You could do so many things if you did not have a dog. You would be free from responsibility and have so much more time for yourself."

But without my dog, what would it matter?

Sparky is His Name

"I will not get another dog," I told anyone who inquired. I had put my seventeen year old companion, Mogul, blind, deaf, and senile, to sleep. He had given me everything and I reciprocated the favor. We had watched over each other's advancing years.

I assured myself now it was time for me. No more dog responsibilities. Walking the dog. Feeding the dog. Loving the dog. Tripping over the water bowl. Now I could travel, go anywhere, come home at any hour, without worrying about someone tending to the dog. It was about time.

A dog was needy, I reminded myself. Dependent. Forty years of dog walking, dog caring, dog dependency. Some dogs had been for the children, some for my husband and me. Now the children were elsewhere and I a widow. It was time for a change.

Without my companion, I noticed certain absences. When I opened the front door, there was no one to greet me. When I ate at the dinner table, there was no one on the floor looking up at me. When I lay in bed at night, there were no footsteps of a dog guarding the house.

I don't know quite how it happened, that two weeks later, I was standing in the animal shelter, that I was staring into the dark pleading eyes of a three month old Lab, that I was picking him up in my arms, that he was smothering my face with kisses, that I was taking him home.

"Why did I do this?" I asked myself as I ran after Sparky while he dug up the backyard, while he discovered the roll of toilet paper, while he ran with a pen in his mouth, while he fled with a cushion, then shredded it, while he retrieved my shoe without my permission, while he opened the mail and then chewed it up, while he jumped high enough to reach the top of the front door and tackled anyone who entered, while he nearly drove to insanity my three cats, while he nibbled, barked, taunted, teased, and quickly chased away every ounce of silence in the house.

"Why did I do this?' I wondered as I tripped over his water bowl, his bones, his football, tennis ball, his favorite rag, and several unknown treasures he had retrieved from the backyard. Daily, I crawled into bed, my legs aching from all the bending and picking up and running after. No longer did I look forward to sitting in the corner of the couch when I watched television. My Lab immediately claimed the spot as his own. From there he could look out onto the street, sleep comfortably at night, and during the day, take his naps and meditate.

In a desperate attempt to regain control of my house, I engaged a trainer. She charged fifty dollars an hour.

"What do you need Sparky to know?" she asked.

"I need him to know he does not have to kiss everyone on the lips, especially when they are standing."

"I need him to know I am walking him down the street, he is not walking me."

"I need him to know it is possible to sit, especially upon command."

Since I had limited funds and since my Lab had other ideas about what he was willing to learn, we settled for the "sit" and the "no" command. Eventually I learned not to take it personally when Sparky chewed up my manuscripts, my pencils, my stuffed bear, and my pillows. I also discovered my dog enjoyed a bone filled with peanut butter, saltine crackers, a treat now and then, and some daily moments of affection. Nothing made his eyes sparkle or tail wag faster then a well-placed hug and a sincere kiss on his cold nose. Sparky learned not to take it personally when I didn't walk as fast as he did, when I didn't throw the ball as many times as he would have liked, and when he wasn't invited to dine with company. He also learned I would not share my meals, my books, my shoes, or my toothpaste. We adjusted.

Sparky soon discovered I wasn't perfect. I realized he wasn't going to make it easy for me. On bad days I resent having to go outside when it's cold, get up early when I want to sleep late, return home for his needs when I am out having a good time, think of him when I want to think of nothing. On his bad days I am certain, he wishes we had more company, that I could run instead of walk, that we shared more adventure, and that he didn't live with three cats.

But we both have so much in common. Sparky needs love as much as I do. He also enjoys companionship. He needs not to feel alone. He requires caring, loyalty, and attention. He appreciates what I have to offer, and I, what he so readily gives.

Sparky doesn't consider me old. With him in my life, neither do I.

The Busybody

"I wish we had a bird," my granddaughter Jenny said one day. She had two cats at her house, one indoor and one outdoor, but no bird. Jenny had big brown eyes that wouldn't let go when she wanted something. Those eyes were directed toward me. "Grandmom, do you want a bird?" she asked hopefully. She knew Grandmom already had box turtles, fish, cats, and a dog. Grandmom's house was full of animals. Why not a bird?

"No Jenny," I told the dark brown eyes, "I don't want a bird. I really do not".

That's what I thought I said. Five minutes later, I found myself in the pet shop with Jenny in hand standing in front of a group of parakeets that were chirping in our direction.

"We're here just to look," I told Jenny firmly. Of course we both knew we just couldn't go out and buy a bird just like that.

But that's exactly what we did. Just like that. Jenny figured it would be wonderful for me to have the bird and she could visit all the time since she lived only ten minutes away. Our bird, the one being put in the box, was white with blue markings. We left the pet shop a short time later with a cage, cuttlebone, bird seed, gravel paper, a mirror, a toy to knock around and a bird bath.

"I don't believe I'm doing this," I kept saying all the way home. But Jenny believed it. In fact, it seemed the most natural thing for us to do. "You see Grandmom" she said with her five year old wisdom, "you are so much better with animals and they all know that and they all keep each other company and they all think you're wonderful and they live forever."

That sounded very nice as we stood in my kitchen, the parakeet in the box, the cats staring at the empty cage, the dog staring at the box. Once the cage was hung in the proper spot against the wall, we named the parakeet Firebird. There was absolutely as much logic to naming the bird as to buying it. Jenny liked the name and that was that.

"Don't worry Grandma," Jenny said. "You just keep it a little while and then I'll take it to my house."

We both knew that would never happen. It was much more fun visiting animals then taking care of them. I had learned that lesson many years ago, when my daughter left her dog with me permanently, when my son left his box turtles with me permanently, and when a few cats here and there wound up in my house permanently though they first belonged to someone else.

After Jenny left, I stood there staring at the bird and he at me. "What am I doing here?" he seemed to ask.

"What are you doing here?" I asked him back.

Neither one of us seemed to know what to do about each other. The dog barked and barked beneath the cage. The cats meowed their complaints beneath the cage. Firebird began to imitate both. It was a cross between a bark and a meow.

"That bird just barked along with the dog," a visitor would comment.

"No, really?" I'd reply.

But I knew of course Firebird did. She became very adept at it.

Firebird had his own mind regarding everything. Even when I put on his cover at night, it wouldn't silence him if he had something to say. I could slip into the kitchen at night trying not to make a noise and Firebird, from beneath the cover, would begin chirping as if it were morning.

I would like to say Firebird and I had a gentle relationship, but it was far from gentle. He would constantly peck at me whenever I cleaned his cage. I would also like to say that the grandchildren all helped take care of him and eventually took him to their house. That never happened. As I write this, Firebird is barking from his cage.

What did happen is that I became accustomed to what Firebird offered. Constant sound. Whenever I walked into the house, there was a greeting from his cage. Whenever I worked in the kitchen doing the dishes, I heard his chatter from behind me. Firebird was a busybody. When the phone rang, he rushed to the side of the cage closest to it and listened in on the conversation, his head cocked to one side. If I washed the floor, he watched me wash it. Setting the table seemed fun to him. He chirped incessantly when I took out the dishes and silverware from the dishwasher..

Firebird made certain the house was never silent.

But more then his constant chatter, I found myself entranced by his busy schedule within the cage. He awoke as soon as the cover came off his cage and immediately set forth in conversation. Usually after he greeted me, he looked into his mirror and made some soft chirping sounds as if to greet himself. Then he had breakfast, took a short nap, and took his bath.

On a sunny day, he bathed with a splash of sun warming him. Then he cleaned himself thoroughly and if there was nothing better to do, took another nap. During the afternoon, he kept busy nibbling at a treat, sharpening his beak, and greeting me whenever I walked into the kitchen. He was very interested in the cats, their movements, and the birds outside the house. He talked to them in the warmer weather when the windows were open.

Always, I felt Firebird's contentment coming from the cage. He greeted each day with energy and anticipation, and yet a certain acceptance, as if he didn't need more then he had. He appeared satisfied with his lot in life.

My world had grown smaller with children no longer running around. Especially in the winter, when the cold and snow kept me inside, I was more aware of my isolation. And then Firebird would chirp from his cage and flutter his wings. He would go about his daily business taking his bath and sunbathing and cleaning his wings, and I would think it didn't matter how small a world was after all.

If one was happy in it.

Napoleon

I have written about starting over before. I wrote about starting over after having cancer. And about starting over as a widow. And when my pets died, I wrote about that starting over also. Each time it was difficult. Sometimes it seemed impossible. But when I was 71years old, my cat Napoleon died, and I wondered if I could ever start over again.

Napoleon was not just a pet. She was my husband's cat. A final link to the past. She was the cat Eph found along with some other kittens, hidden behind a trash can, clinging to her protective mother. He rushed into the house, and surprised me with the words, for he was not a cat lover, "You wouldn't believe the beautiful kitten I just found. White hair and blue eyes." Napoleon was on the bottom of four kittens, curled together to keep warm. We took two, a brother and sister. Eph named both after his heroes, Winston (Churchill) and Napoleon. Winston passed on two years before, but it was Napoleon who represented the past. She was the cat whose blue eyes never left our faces when we entered the house we had just moved into at the shore. She was the cat who sat with us when the roof leaked, when the hurricanes tested our endurance. And when Eph no longer had the energy of a young man, she was the cat who lay on his bed, her wise eyes comforting him more than any person could.

This time I did not grow angry as I had when cancer attacked my body. Or frightened and unable to function when widowhood descended upon me. Though I wept like a child when I found out Napoleon could not be saved, though I consoled myself that she had lived a long life of 15 years, I felt like a traveler suddenly losing her way on the road she had journeyed for a long time. There did not seem to be a reason to begin again with another pet. I had a dog and a cat remaining. There was a parakeet chirping in a cage and two box turtles staring at me from the tank. I did not feel confident the old solutions would work, replacing one pet with another.

And suddenly, my age became a factor. Did I have a right to take on another young life? A sore hip here, a wounded spirit there. Sometimes I even needed help to get my pets to a veterinarian.

And so I told my friends that I was finished adding pets to my household. How often can one start over, I asked them, and was it worth it? In fact, when I thought about it, I told anyone who had the patience to listen, love seemed the villain. How painless life would be without it.

Or so I thought for a short while. Until the responses arrived. From friends who had lost pets. And who had lost loved ones. Friends older than I and younger than I. Friends who had loved their dogs and birds and cats and spouses and companions. Friends who reminded me that loving is the privilege, the gift, the energy of life. Worth the pain. Worth anything it might cost. And that loving a pet was a rehearsal for loving one another. No matter what our age. One woman who rescued cats told me she had given an 87 year old woman a two year old cat. "No one is too old to love," she said.

"I heard you lost Napoleon," a neighbor said as she entered my home shortly after, and hugged me. And the words arrived, I somehow knew would come one day. "I have four kittens born a few weeks ago," she continued, her blue eyes asking if I was ready. "And one is so ugly. Very smart. But ugly."

You are intelligent readers. So you already know that I answered without hesitation. "I'll take the ugly one."

I named her Beauty.

Sweetcake's Revenge

She showed up one day at my front door, just lying there on my welcome mat. As if she had read the message and took it literally. Pure white with a brown tail and brown bits about her kittenish face. Her beauty captured me.

For days she did not miss a meal set outside on the porch. She would eat, clean herself, then thank me by rubbing her body against my legs. She never forgot her "thank you." But she would not allow me to pet her. She seemed terrified of everything that moved. Always looking over her shoulder. Turning around quickly at the sound of a car or a person walking down the street. Or the bark of a dog. There were so many things to be frightened of in her outside world and she seemed fearful of all of them. Most wild cats were accustomed to their rough life, but this cat appeared new to the outside and didn't know how to handle it. I understood her fearfulness for I also was afraid. As a single older woman with many responsibilities, I too found myself often looking over my shoulder for the next crises.

She had the sweetest face I had ever seen on a cat, and so I named her Sweetcake, even before I trapped her in a cage, took her to the veterinarian, had her altered so she would not produce kittens, gave her the necessary shots, and brought her inside my home..

Then the nightmare began. How could I have been so wrong in naming her, I would think during the next year? Where had the sweet cat gone and how was she replaced by this unloving, unaffectionate aloof cat that had come to live in my house? She would not let me pick her up, pet her, or give her any sign of affection. She would not even remain in the room I was in for more than a few moments. Wherever I walked, Sweetcake would flee as if I were the enemy. She had little to do with the other cats or the dog. It was as if they did not exist in her world. And her final revenge against all of us were her "accidents." On the couch. On the chair. Wherever I, or my dog or the other two cats napped, Sweetcake's urine became the familiar aroma there and everywhere else. The animals avoided Sweetcake and the areas she visited.

Guests had plenty to say about Sweetcake. "Why don't you just get rid of her?" they asked as they settled uncomfortably on a plastic cover. "You can't live this way forever, with that cat ruining all the furniture."

But I knew getting rid of her would not be so simple. No one would take her with such an offensive habit. If I put her back outside again, which I thought of more than I would have liked to admit, she would not survive long. And then there were my own selfish reasons for keeping her. As an older adult, I feared the exciting challenges in my life were over. I needed to know I could still dare to do what many around me now considered impossible. Turn Sweetcake into a loving well-behaved housecat.

I kept hoping for a change in behavior. Kitty litter pans were placed in strategic places to make it easier for her. She seemed to like the small red one in the hallway. I bought her two of them. They worked for awhile and then she would return to her old habit. There were times after one of her accidents that she would look at me with a haughtiness as if she were showing me just who was boss. Her name became a bitter reminder of the mistake I had made when I added her to my inside cat population. I knew I was reaching the end of my patience.

One day after months of frustration, I lay resting on the bed, the cat brush still in my hand. My older cat had just enjoyed her grooming time. Sweetcake often watched as I brushed the other cats but never allowed it to be done to her. This time, slowly, she crept toward me and the hand that held the brush. I did not dare move a muscle as she moved forward until her head rested on the brush. She looked up at me in that moment of decision and I knew how she felt. "We can't go on like this forever," I gently told her. "It's got to come to an end." Perhaps Sweetcake was thinking the same thing. Maybe finally after all the months of offering her my home, my understanding and my love, she decided she could trust me. She pushed her head into the brush, turned her body upside down, paws in the air, encouraging me to stroke one side and then another. She purred beneath the brush, her expression one of rapture as if she had been waiting for such an experience for a very long time. From that brushing on, Sweetcake became a different cat. She sleeps with me and now and then crawls beneath my hand to be stroked. But only on her terms. And she plays with the other cats as if she has finally decided to join the family. But more important, Sweetcake stopped having her "accidents".

She found the strength to overcome her fears. And with Sweetcake leading the way, I feel I can also.

The Outdoor Gang

I call the outside couch on my porch "The Bed and Breakfast" because there is always a guest cat beneath it, waiting for a meal and a good night's sleep.

Aside from my indoor cats, there are always outside cats at my house. There must be someone directing the cat population. Somewhere there is a sign that reads, "Just walk two blocks down the street, turn to the right, find the white house, and you'll get a good meal and a saucer of something good to drink." Sometimes I think there is a "cat newspaper" with a classified section advertising my front porch and the shelter it provides. Because they always show up. A black and white cat with a pathetic face. A bright orange one who looks as if he hasn't been fed in weeks. A tabby cat pregnant and tired from carrying her litter.

They come and they go, these outdoor cats. Some stay for a longer time then others. I try to trap them and have them neutered, so the cat population won't explode in our neighborhood. Neighbors tell me the reason the cats find me is because they know there will be food on my porch for a tired traveler. They tell me if I take away the food, the cats will also leave. Now how could I do that? Knowing an animal was hungry or looking for shelter on the outside? How could I sleep at night beneath my warm blankets knowing this? Especially in the winter, when the snows come and food is difficult to find.

There have been dozens of strays passing by through the years. We have an understanding with each other. They can stay as long as they like. They must share with any other cat on the porch. Troublemakers are not welcome.

Gray was the outdoor cat that remained with me the longest. He showed up one day as a kitten, on the back steps. He had this expression on his face that made it clear from the start, he wasn't going anywhere for a long time. And he didn't. Not for eight years.

Every day I would open the back door and Gray, I called him Gray because that was his color from nose to tail, was perched on the back steps waiting for his meal. He would also show up at night because he expected two meals a day, with something good in a saucer to drink. I called him by his name and he always snapped to attention, turning my way in recognition.

Gray mysteriously vanished during the winter for a month or so. I assumed he had another home where he was more comfortable during the cold weather. One winter, he disappeared and never returned. With outdoor cats, there is always the danger of being hit by a car or straying too far, and not being able to find the way back. I always kept that in mind. There was a limit to my attachment to an outdoor cat because there were no guarantees that he would return. Although after so many years, I felt Gray had become part of my family.

About a year later, I was walking down the street about five blocks from my house. A gray cat sat on someone's step, staring at me. He looked very much like Gray and as if he belonged where he was sitting.

"Gray?" I called.

The head snapped up at attention. For a moment the cat came forward. Then he hesitated, and returned to his former location. If it was Gray, he had decided he had found something better. I was now part of his past.

Different cats arrive every day. Some belong to other people who let them roam about the neighborhood. I feed them anyway. Some are tired and just need shelter for a night or two. Each seems to have a story to tell, but many are too tired to tell it.

"Is there food for me?" they seem to ask.

"Of course," I say. "Eat well and go on your way when you are ready."

The strays have an understanding among each other. If one is eating, the other waits patiently. If one is impatient and selfish, there is some spitting and loud meowing to put him in place. Now and then they bring an offering of gratitude and leave it at my doorstep as a thank you. A dead mouse, or bird. I understand its significance and that a cat can't curb his hunter's instinct.

When one feeds outdoor cats, as I do, it becomes an expense, sometimes one that I can't easily afford. There are organizations out there that do what they can to ease the cost. One woman named Mary, from such an organization, left bags of food on my porch when she found out I had four outdoor cats to feed at one time. She also paid to have the cats neutered, and to have their shots. I was amazed to find out the work Mary did, that when she learned of a starving cat, or homeless one, or abused one, she would try to track it down, save it, give it a future in the environment. Gentle people they are whose lives are devoted to helping strays survive. While other people are sitting at dinner tables after work, many of these devoted lovers of animals are leaving food out in cat stations where stray cats gather. They also take sick cats home so that they might recover and regain their dignity. It is a constant vigilance because many people do not neuter their cats, nor do they care what happens to them in the outside world.

I was shocked to learn from Mary that 2 cats can have an average of 2–3 litters per year with an average of 4 kittens per litter. Left unfixed and counting the original cats and all of their offspring and their offspring's offspring total about 100,000 cats in ten years. There are approximately 60 million strays in the United States alone. If every family just had one cat fixed, we would be in much better shape with the outdoor gang.

Beginning Again

New beginnings are like getting ready for an exciting trip to a place you've never been before. Or like falling in love without a parachute. There is always the promise of adventure and none of the security of knowing the outcome.

When my 12-year-old cat had a stroke and died, my grown children suggested I get a kitten. I was uncertain whether I was ready for this new beginning. No matter how tempting the journey, for the first time in all my years of loving pets, I wasn't certain that I should continue bringing animals into my life.

Though I still had my five-year-old dog, another 12-year-old cat and a parakeet living in a cage in the kitchen, it occurred to me that perhaps I was being selfish at my age, adding another animal to my family. When I'd adopted a pet in my thirties, I was confident that I would outlive him. But now, at more than twice that age, my certainty had disappeared. Chances were the animal might outlive me. And then what? I had never thought of the future in these terms before, and did not enjoy thinking like this now.

There were other reasons for not introducing a new pet into the house. I told myself, "Be reasonable. Be practical. There are benefits to keeping the pet population down. Less work emptying kitty litter. Less money spent for pet food. Fewer trips to the veterinarian. When the one cat remaining is gone, that will be the end of it. No more cats. Eventually no more pets. And then you will have more freedom."

I knew it was good advice, but the house took on shadows I never noticed before. And a stillness that seemed ominous. There had always been two and sometimes three or four inside cats. Now, the one remaining cat, who had daily groomed the other, slept with her paws wrapped around a stuffed animal. Something was missing from her life and she knew it. The dog, who had been a loving companion to his deceased cat friend, appeared listless. Bored. His nap times increased. And so did mine.

Yes, it was easier now. Too easy. I lay in bed one day, persuading myself to remain there another hour and another. In fact, when I piled up all the sad stories I could think of and all the pets I had bid good-by, I thought it would be quite easy to remain in bed the entire day. After all, what did the outside world offer? Trouble, that's what. If I didn't go out, why even bother to get dressed? Who would know anyway, if I walked the dog in my long coat?

"You need a kitten," my daughter told me one day as she frowned in my direction, sensing my mood. "This place needs some excitement."

That's how Sunny came to live here. A tiny thing rescued from the woods, he arrived in my daughter's arms, rehabilitated, cleaned, de-fleaed, and inoculated. "He's perfect for you," she said. I had not yet reached that conclusion. Neither had Sunny.

It took only a second for him to step on to the living room rug, but in that moment, silence rushed from my home—exiting through the front door—and chaos entered without warning.

The dog ran after the kitten. The older cat hissed and spit. The two ganged up on the new kid in town. *What ingratitude*, I thought. Here I'd been concerned that they were lonely, in deep depression, and they were rejecting my solution.

"I'm too old for this," I said at one point in the evening, as I tried to catch the kitten that had hidden in the basement.

"I'm too old for this," I repeated after four trips to the basement, two stiff knees kneeling on the kitchen floor, two attempts to scramble beneath the bed to retrieve a frightened Sunny hiding from the dog that was on guard duty.

Exhausted and certain I had made a mistake, I pleaded, "Take him back. I'm too old for this," as soon as my daughter entered the house the next day.

At that moment, I meant it. I believed it.

I stood in the kitchen, tears in my eyes. I was crying not only for the cat in my mind already gone, but for the part of me that had vanished also.

My enthusiasm to try something new. The belief that I could. The energy to do it.

I wanted everyone who told me I *was* young enough, to be here, running after this kitten. I wanted them to be with me at 5:00 in the morning when Sunny arose and decided to attack my feet beneath the covers and then wake up all the other animals in the house. I wanted them here when he explored the lamp shade until he knocked over the lamp, or decided everything on the kitchen table needed reorganizing, removing all napkins, spoons, glasses filled with water, and of course any tempting food on the plates that begged to be shared.

But I knew I could not blame it all on Sunny. It was just too difficult to begin again. To love again. To take on the responsibility again. I was frightened because I did not know if I had it in me. I didn't want to find out.

While I agonized over his future, Sunny had settled in a basket and was enjoying a nap. The sun settled on his beige fur. The old cat had left her stuffed animals to sit by the basket, suddenly interested in the new member of our family. The dog, exhausted from kitten guard duty, had settled in the same sunny spot, sharing it. It was as if they understood things had changed. Nothing would ever be the same. Something had left and something else had entered. Now they would have to adjust. I understood the message in their eyes. We could do it together, accept the change, and perhaps even enjoy the challenge of beginning again—if I let myself.

The next morning, Sunny investigated the kitchen with renewed interest. Something was different and he noticed it immediately: it was raining for the first time since he had come to live with me. The raindrops splattered on the roof and made tantalizing sounds. He looked up as he explored each room. As if he expected whatever he heard to eventually come down and introduce itself. They were just raindrops falling. But their sound was new to him. And suddenly, through his eyes, the falling rain became refreshingly wondrous for me, too.

I hurried to get dressed. Sunny started his adventures early, and I didn't want to miss any of them.

A Reminder

Writing about squirrels might not be everyone's choice, but it is often mine. I do not think there is anything more beautiful today than the four squirrels silhouetted against the sky. As usual, they are sitting in my tree. The tree is tall with many limbs stretching into the blueness above. Each squirrel is on a limb, very high up. As I look at them, they look at me. Neither of us knows what the other is thinking. And yet we both know we want to survive the day.

Each morning I toss whatever leftovers I have out my side bedroom window. Sometimes it is potatoes, sometimes carrots. Stale bread. Spaghetti. Much to my surprise they like spaghetti. They seem not to be fussy about their menu. And they are always hungry. I do not like to waste food, so they make me feel much better about the dinner I cannot finish or the bread not eaten up quickly enough. Whatever is left, I feed to the squirrels.

I have even been known to take leftovers from others. Only those I know well. Only those who will not look at me strangely when I say, "Don't throw all that away. Just put it in a baggie and I'll take it home for the squirrels." I must admit I do this often in restaurants with food left on my plate, but they are accustomed to their diners taking their leftovers home.

There are usually four of them. Perhaps they are family. They come from down the block. The squirrels hear my window open from wherever they are and then I see them rushing toward me. They travel from tree to tree. They do not want to be late for breakfast. I am always amazed at the gracefulness of them, balancing themselves on the thinnest of limbs, never missing a jump, and then to the roof next door and over it and finally to the tallest limbs of my tree. I wish my aged limbs could be so agile.

And then it is down to business. At first they scurry about chasing each other, in competition for what there is to eat. Afraid there will not be enough for all. This one chases that one back up the tree. Then down they come, one after the other. Finally, through good sense, they decide no one is going to get to eat this way. And so one at a time, they pick up a piece of whatever has been offered, and carrying it in their mouths, they travel quickly to a safe place in the tree. They sit on back paws, holding their treasure in their front ones and they seem almost human dining there. Their bushy tails shake in excitement as they devour their prizes. Then back down for more. Traveling upside down. Hanging in impossible positions. Almost defying gravity. Occasionally they will pause, look over at me, I am certain, with appreciation, then back to inspecting what remains on the ground.

I spend many moments just watching them. There is much for me to do but it can wait. There is also much for me to cope with in the day coming up. In my world and in the larger one. But that can wait also. How I begin my day is important for it will influence how I look at my day. The squirrels remind me how simple life can be, if I allow it.

Soon the squirrels will move on. They will disappear into the backyard and go about their mysterious lives. I will probably not recognize them even if they happen to visit again while I am taking my morning walk. For I only know them when they are in my tall tree. Then they become part of my life.

And for some reason, make mine better.

Each New Day

It is a new day but I do not want to begin. There is no eagerness to start the morning. I think of all the reasons why I should remain in bed, beneath the blankets. Fear can do that to a person. Depression can also. Giving up is a good reason to remain in bed and ignore the new day.

My dog does not allow me to surrender to my mood. He is the first to tell me it is a new day. He does not need a clock to know when each new day arrives. He stands at the side of the bed. I feel his presence. I hear his breathing. Slowly, I open my eyes. "It's a new day," he says through excited eyes and a wagging tail. I hear his thoughts. "Come on. Let's see what it holds. I've got to get out in that backyard and check out things that might have happened during the night. Perhaps the next door neighbor will toss me a nice meat bone today. Or you'll play ball with me. You never can tell what's going to happen, but it's got to be good." His ears stand at attention. He thinks only fun will come today. He does not have any doubts, or fears regarding the hours ahead. They can only be wonderful. And when I look at his eager expression and feel his energy, I begin to think so also.

The two cats soon follow. They softly creep about my bed, traveling slowly to my shoulders. They stare into my eyes. "So, how about it," they seem to say. "It's a new day. We can start all over. We can begin again. Come on. Get up. We're hungry. Then we can deal with the everyday things. You're a fighter. Get up and fight." Cats carry a silent wisdom. They will cope with whatever the day brings. They immediately sit on a window ledge to observe the arriving dawn. Later, they will have breakfast, and then take their nap. They do that each new day. Today, they bring the first smile to my face.

As I lay there, I turn toward the window and catch the first few slivers of daylight. Usually, there is something about a new day that excites me.

Even though I might have appointments that I am not looking forward to keeping, even though my body parts get cranky thinking of what they must do, when I see that sunrise each day, I feel a gift has been given, wrapped and delivered especially to me. But today I feel a shadow cast across the sunrise. And I am having trouble removing it.

Just then I hear my parakeet call to me, as it does each morning about this time. I walk into the kitchen. The parakeet says hello. "Hello," I reply. "It's a new day," she tells me in her way. "I'm singing to brighten the morning. How do you like my song? I sing a new song each new day. Now how about giving me my bath. And a cheerful good morning might be due me. It can't be a bad day if you've got a song." I cannot disagree. I hum a tune as I feed the bird. Then I open the shades and look outside. The outdoor stray cat is sitting on the porch couch staring up at me, waiting. "Good morning," he nods, his expression telling me, "I've been out here all night guarding the house. Waiting for the new day. I can't wait to see what adventures are before me. Is there anything good that I can eat coming from your house this morning? And by the way, you have nothing to worry about. Not with me out here." There is expectation in his eyes. I do not disappoint him. A hearty breakfast is delivered. Seeing the cat devour it, gives me an appetite for my own first meal of the day.

As I stand there, the sun opens up wide on the morning and splashes across the street. "Nothing can stop me unless I let it," it speaks to me through its sunlight. "My light will chase away the darkness and the fear. No one will rob me of today."

I rush inside to get dressed, my energy suddenly renewed by all the life forces surrounding me. No one will rob me of this day, either.

One More Thought

You have met my pet companions, some as they came into my life, some as they left. But this is an ongoing story, for I never know who will show up tomorrow or how they will affect my life. They might come to remain a lifetime, or just for a quick visit. A cat might be waiting on my porch tonight, sent there by another.

"You will always get a meal and a bowl of water. You can count on it," this cat will be told, for the animal community is aware of such drop-ins and spreads the word. Otherwise how would so many know my address?

Somehow, they always find me, and I find them. Each one is different. Each fighting to survive with as much dignity as possible. Each asking little and giving much.

They heap their gifts upon me. Generosity. Affection. Understanding. Acceptance. And the greatest gift of all. Their unconditional love.

Essays appearing in Chicken Soup for the Soul Series

✦

By Harriet May Savitz

Chicken Soup for the Grandma's Soul

A Grandmother Again

A Day at Grandmom's House

Jenny's Antique

Chicken Soup for the Soul of America

Beep if You Love America

Neighbors Knowing Neighbors

We Are One (Promotional Material)

Chicken Soup for the Golden Soul

Strike Out or Home Run

Chicken Soup for the Sports Fan's Soul

Strike Out or Home Run

Chicken Soup for the Cat Lover's Soul

Beginning Again

Chicken Soup for the Grandparent's Soul

Somewhere Babe Ruth Is Smiling

Chicken Soup for the Girlfriend's Soul

The Artist's Chair

Chicken Soup for the Kid's Soul 2

The Measuring Line (with Beth Savitz Laliberte)

Chicken Soup for the Soul—Celebrating Mothers & Daughters

I Am Ready

Chicken Soup for the Mother and Son Soul

The Yellow Boat

Chicken Soup for the Sister's Soul 2

I Do Have Sisters

Chicken Soup for the Beach Lover's Soul

Only at the Beach

Confessions of a Jersey Girl

Four Blocks Up

Chicken Soup for the Working Mom's Soul

A Privilege

Chicken Soup—Life Lessons for Busy Moms

Busy Bees

Chicken Soup for the Soul Celebrates Grandmothers

Jenny's Antique

Really Alive

Chicken Soup for the Recovering Soul

Creating My Own Recovery

Chicken Soup for the Soul-Recipes for Busy Moms

The Latkes Epidemic

2008
Chicken Soup for the Soul Celebrating People
Who Make a Difference—The Headlines You'll Never Read

The Wall

Chicken Soup for the Soul—Love Stories

The New Odd Couple

Chicken Soup for the Soul—A Tribute to Mom

Not Just on Mother's Day

A Mother First

A Good Call

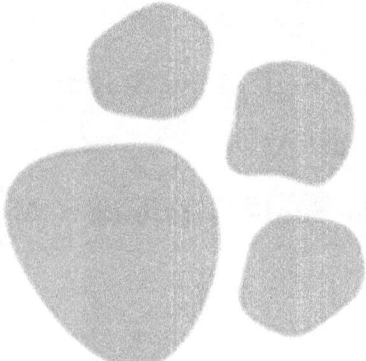

About the Author

Harriet May Savitz has over 24 books published by major publishers. Savitz's book, "Run, Don't Walk," was made into an ABC Afterschool Special produced by Henry Winkler. Her book, "Fly, Wheels, Fly," was nominated for the Dorothy Canfield Fisher Award. Her young adult novel, "The Lionhearted," was listed as one of the most popular books in The University of Iowa's Books for Young Adults. She received the PSLA 1981 Outstanding Pennsylvania Author Award and in celebration of the International Year of Disabled Persons, received recognition for her nonfiction young adult book, "Wheelchair Champions."

www.harrietmaysavitz.com
hmaysavitz@aol.com

Credits: Contributor to 20 Chicken Soup of the Soul books ... Chocolate for a Woman's Courage (Chocolate Series-Fireside Books) Modern Maturity..Mature Years ..Asbury Park Press ... Boomer Times & Senior News ... Various newspapers around the country ... King Features Syndicate.. .24 Published Books ... an ABC Afterschool Special produced by Henry Winkler of book, "Run, Don't Walk." essays appearing in newspapers and magazines.... "Messages From Somewhere—Inspiring Stories of Life After 60" (Publishers Weekly—2/18/02—Midwest Book Review 5–02—Little Treasure Publisher) PSLA 1981 Outstanding Pennsylvania Author Award (Pennsylvania School Library Association Award) Others books of Essays—"More Than Ever—A View From My 70s" "Hello Grandparents Wherever You Are" (authorhouse.com) "Keeping It Going—After 70 & Before" (Author House.com) Children's Picture Book—"Is A Worry Worrying You" co-authored Ferida Wolff—(Tanglewood Books-2005) The Story Book co-authored Ferida Wolff—Andersen/Random House (spring-2008)

Children's and young adult books have been reissued by Authors-Guild/iUniverse

978-0-595-50251-6
0-595-50251-2